T0269166

SpringerBriefs in Statistics

More information about this series at http://www.springer.com/series/8921

Joaquim Pinto da Costa

Rankings and Preferences

New Results in Weighted Correlation
and Weighted Principal Component
Analysis with Applications

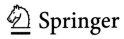 Springer

Joaquim Pinto da Costa
Department of Mathematics
University of Porto
Porto
Portugal

ISSN 2191-544X ISSN 2191-5458 (electronic)
SpringerBriefs in Statistics
ISBN 978-3-662-48343-5 ISBN 978-3-662-48344-2 (eBook)
DOI 10.1007/978-3-662-48344-2

Library of Congress Control Number: 2015950035

Springer Heidelberg New York Dordrecht London

Printed on acid-free paper

Springer-Verlag GmbH Berlin Heidelberg is part of Springer Science+Business Media
(www.springer.com)

To my mother
Maria Pinto de Castro

Preface

This book concerns weighted correlation and applications involving rankings and preferences. For instance, recommendation of data analysis tools, stock trading support, information retrieval, meta-learning, and recommender systems. Instead of using Spearman's rank correlation coefficient, which is not suitable in some applications, some weighted correlation coefficients will be presented and analyzed in the book and will then be used in a number of applications. The first of these coefficients, r_W, was proposed by us in 2001 [61, 63, 93] and it weighs the distance between two ranks using a linear function of those ranks, giving more importance to higher ranks than lower ones. The statistical distribution of r_W together with some motivating applications will be the subject of Chap. 2.

In Chap. 3 another weighted rank correlation coefficient, r_{W2}, introduced in [74] and applied in a bioinformatics context in [73], will be presented. This coefficient is the second of its series, following the coefficient r_W which was motivated by a machine learning problem concerning the recommendation of learning algorithms. Unlike Spearman's r_S, which treats all ranks equally, these coefficients weigh the distance between two ranks using a linear function of those ranks in the case of r_W and a quadratic function in the case of r_{W2}. The presence of ties, which can happen naturally in some of the applications, will also be taken into consideration in Chap. 3, together with a simulation study to compare the three coefficients r_{W2}, r_W and r_S.

In Chap. 4 we describe in the first part the new developments in weighted Principal Component Analysis (PCA) [42] and in the second part a new method to select variables. The focus is on problems where the values taken by each variable do not all have the same importance and where the data may be contaminated with noise and contain outliers, as is the case with microarray data. This kind of data, which contains the expression levels of a large number of genes (variables), measured simultaneously, for a relatively much smaller number of tissue samples, presents many statistical challenges. There we propose the use of a weighted correlation coefficient, as an alternative to Pearsons, leading thus to a so-called weighted PCA (WPCA1). Then, we apply WPCA1 to the problem of analysing gene expression datasets. In the second part of Chap. 4 we propose a new

PCA-based algorithm to iteratively select the most important genes in a microarray dataset. We show that this algorithm produces better results when WPCA1 is used instead of the usual PCA. We also show that this algorithm used together with support vector machines can compete with the significance analysis of microarrays (SAM) supervised algorithm [97, 98].

Another weighted Principal Component Analysis (WPCA2) for time series data, is presented in Chap. 5. First, in some situations the number of observations in each series is too large and so it is of paramount importance to be able to compress the series, thus reducing its dimension. Second, in a time series context, it is frequent that some observation times are more important than others and the usual PCA cannot take this into account. Thus, a weighted PCA specific for time series data, which was introduced in [70], is described in this chapter and then applied to well-known datasets.

In Chap. 6 we will describe a method for the weighted clustering of time series. This method does not give the same importance to all the observations; instead, it lets the most important observations, for instance the most recent, have a larger weight. A fundamental problem in the clustering of time series is the choice of a relevant metric, and in this chapter, we will use a metric, based on Pearson correlation coefficient, which uses the notion of weighted mean and weighted covariance. We present also some motivating applications.

Finally, we thank everyone who has collaborated with us in the subject of weighted correlation and applications and in particular Pavel Brazdil, Carlos Soares, and Luís Roque. We thank also the editor Eva Hiripi.

Porto   Joaquim Pinto da Costa
January 2015

Contents

Chapter 1
Introduction

Abstract The main motivation underlying this book consists in applications involving rankings, like for instance preferences stated by humans, recommendation of data analysis tools, stock trading support, information retrieval, meta-learning and recommender systems. For the evaluation of the different methods, the comparisons of different rankings by means of an appropriate, weighted, correlation coefficient is used. Some weighted correlation coefficients will be presented and analyzed in the book. We will also present some interesting applications like for instance in bioinformatics, principal component analysis, and clustering.

1.1 Some Motivating Applications

The motivation underlying this work applies to a broad range of applications involving rankings. For instance, rankings of alternatives representing the preferences stated by humans or recommendations provided by decision support systems. A general application, which was our first motivation, is the evaluation of methods to predict rankings. Such methods exist in a variety of situations like the recommendation of data analysis tools, stock trading support (i.e., ranking of a set of stocks), information retrieval, recommender systems, and user preferences. From these, information retrieval [53] and recommender systems [87] are two areas where rankings are already widely used. Other areas where it may be advantageous to use a ranking approach, rather than the usual supervised classification, are medicine (e.g., diagnosis of an illness or choice of an adequate test or treatment) and control systems (e.g., choice of the correct action to carry out).

One of the first applications that have been considered and that was indeed one of the motivations to develop weighted correlation coefficients comes from the field of machine learning; more precisely, meta-learning: given a certain number of algorithms to perform a given task, one would like to rank those algorithms from 1, the most adequate, to n, the worst. Then, if we have more than one method to rank the algorithms, we have to evaluate the quality of all of the methods in order to choose the best ranking method. To do that, we have to concentrate on problems where the true ranking of all of the algorithms is known, and then we compare that

© The Author(s) 2015
J. Pinto da Costa, *Rankings and Preferences*,
SpringerBriefs in Statistics, DOI 10.1007/978-3-662-48344-2_1

true ranking with the rankings provided by every ranking method. This comparison is usually done by means of a correlation coefficient like Spearman's r_S. Nevertheless, in Spearman's coefficient, all ranks are given the same importance. However, in this application of ranking algorithms, the user starts by using the first algorithms suggested by the method and if there is enough time and resources, tries all of the algorithms; otherwise no. It is thus clear that the algorithms in the top positions are far more important than those in the last positions, but Spearman's coefficient is not sensitive to that. In fact, rather surprisingly, rank importance is rarely taken into account [40]. Similar remarks can also be made concerning the area of recommender systems [14].

Another example which also involves rankings generated by models and rankings representing human preferences, is given in [9], where the authors investigate methods to infer user preferences concerning health profiles and have used Spearman's r_S to assess performance. However, it is common knowledge that when stating their preference as rankings, humans rank the most preferred alternatives, i.e., the ones ranked at the top, more accurately than the others, and so r_S is not really appropriate. Many other examples could be given, like for instance in the area of bioinformatics, which, as we will see later, is a privileged application in this book.

Given that ranking is a learning task different from existing ones, like classification, regression, or clustering, it requires different evaluation procedures. This evaluation was indeed the driving force for the development of weighted correlation coefficients [61, 63, 67, 93].

1.2 Weighted Correlation and Applications

This book is devoted to correlation, more precisely weighted correlation, and applications. A common rank correlation coefficient is Spearman's, which is not a weighted measure but was nevertheless our starting point to develop weighted coefficients. There has been a growing interest about weighted measures of rank correlation [10, 61, 63, 74, 81, 92, 93]; that is, measures that, unlike Spearman's [94] coefficient which treat all ranks equally, weigh ranks by choosing a suitable weight function. For example, by using weights proportionally to how high the ranks are, as will be seen in the applications, although other types of weight functions could be considered. We will start by making a brief introduction to correlation and apply Spearman's rank correlation coefficient to a particular problem, motivating thus the need for a weighted measure.

The objective of correlation coefficients is to assess the degree of monotonicity between two or more series of paired data. By monotonicity, we mean a tendency for the values in the series to increase or decrease together (positive correlation) or for one to increase as the other decreases (negative correlation). They are applicable to paired data, i.e., data where there is some connection between corresponding members of the samples.

Rank correlation coefficients are less restrictive than other methods, e.g., Pearson's correlation coefficient, because they do not try to fit one particular kind of relationship, linear or other, to the data. They achieve this by using the ranks of the sample values rather than the values themselves. To use these coefficients, we must first rank the observations in each sample, X and Y, from 1 (highest rank) to n (lowest rank), where n is the number of pairs of observations. We thus obtain $r(X_i)$ and $r(Y_i)$ where X_i and Y_i are the pair of values corresponding to observation i in each sample and $r(X_i)$ $(r(Y_i))$ returns the rank of value i in the first series (second series). For sake of simplicity, we will use frequently the ranks directly rather than the values in the series. That is, $R_i = r(X_i)$ and $Q_i = r(Y_i)$. One interesting fact about rank correlation is that, contrary to other correlation methods, it can be used not only on numerical data but on any data that can be ranked. An example of the use of such methods is the analysis of sales data where the aim is to assess whether there is correlation between marketing activities (i.e., visits to clients) and the number of sales [57, Chap. 9].

Weighted correlation is concerned with the use of weights assigned to the subjects in the calculation of a correlation coefficient between two variables X and Y [74]. The weights can either be naturally available beforehand or chosen by the user to serve a specific purpose. For instance, if there is a different number of measurements on each subject, it is natural to use these numbers as weights and calculate the correlation between the subject means. On the other hand, if the variables X and Y represent, for instance, the ranks of preferences of two human beings over a set of n items, one might want to give larger weights to the first preferences, as these are more accurate.

Suppose in a general context that (X_i, Y_i) is the pair of values corresponding to observation i in each sample and p_i the weight attributed to this observation, such that $\sum_{i=1}^{n} p_i = 1$. Then, a sample weighted correlation coefficient is given by the formula,

$$
\begin{aligned}
r_p &= \frac{\sum_{i=1}^{n} p_i (X_i - \overline{X}_p)(Y_i - \overline{Y}_p)}{\sqrt{\sum_{i=1}^{n} p_i (X_i - \overline{X}_p)^2}\sqrt{\sum_{i=1}^{n} p_i (Y_i - \overline{Y}_p)^2}} \\
&= \frac{\sum_{i=1}^{n} p_i X_i Y_i - \sum_{i=1}^{n} p_i X_i \sum_{i=1}^{n} p_i Y_i}{\sqrt{\sum_{i=1}^{n} p_i X_i^2 - (\sum_{i=1}^{n} p_i X_i)^2}\sqrt{\sum_{i=1}^{n} p_i Y_i^2 - (\sum_{i=1}^{n} p_i Y_i)^2}},
\end{aligned} \tag{1.1}
$$

where $\overline{X}_p = \sum_{i=1}^{n} p_i X_i$ and $\overline{Y}_p = \sum_{i=1}^{n} p_i Y_i$ are the weighted means. When all of the p_i are equal they cancel out, giving the usual formula for the Pearson's product-moment correlation coefficient.

In this book, we present new correlation coefficients, weighted correlation coefficients, that are applicable to problems where the correlation between two series of paired data is affected by the importance of each data value. For instance, lower values or lower ranks (in the case of rank correlation) are more important than larger ranks and, thus, distance in lower ranks should have larger impact on the correlation coefficient.

In order to illustrate the need for weighted measures of correlation, let us now
consider the following problem concerning the relevance of a set of n documents to
a particular subject. Suppose that $\mathbf{R} = (R_1, R_2, \ldots, R_n)$, represents the ranking of a
set of n documents determined by an expert user in terms of the relevance to a given
query. Suppose further that Q_i, $i = 1, \ldots, n$, represents the ranking of the same set
of documents provided by a search engine, given the same query. The quality of the
output of the search engine in this particular situation (i.e., this query) can be assessed
by measuring the similarity or concordance between the two rankings. However, top-
ranked documents are more important than those that are ranked lower, because the
probability that the user will analyze the former is higher. Thus, the quality of the
output is more affected by the similarity at the top of the rankings rather than at the
bottom.

Rank correlation coefficients such as Spearman's [57, 94, Chap. 9] can be used
to quantify the similarity between two rankings. However, Spearman's coefficient
treats all ranks equally and is, therefore, not entirely suitable for applications such
as the one just described. In order to illustrate this, let us consider the following
situation where we have not one but two search engines. As said, $\mathbf{R}$ represents the
ranking of a set of n documents determined by an expert. Similarly, let now $\mathbf{Q}$ and
$\mathbf{Z}$ represent the ranking of the same set of documents provided by two competing
search engines for the same query (Table 1.1). We want now to decide which of the
two search engines gives better results for this query. Now, the quality of the two
rankings $\mathbf{Q}$ and $\mathbf{Z}$ can be evaluated by calculating their correlation to ranking $\mathbf{R}$,
using Spearman's coefficient. A priori, the one with higher Spearman's correlation
is the best.

Table 1.1 Three rankings of ten documents for a given query: $\mathbf{R}$ represents the relevance for the
query, and $\mathbf{Q}$ and $\mathbf{Z}$ represent two rankings obtained from different search engines for the same
query

Doc. (i)	Ranks			$(R_i - Q_i)^2$	$(R_i - Z_i)^2$
	R_i	Q_i	Z_i		
D1	1	2	3	1	4
D2	2	1	5	1	9
D3	3	4	2	1	1
D4	4	6	1	4	9
D5	5	5	6	0	1
D6	6	3	4	9	4
D7	7	8	7	1	0
D8	8	9	8	1	0
D9	9	10	9	1	0
D10	10	7	10	9	0

Now, to calculate Spearman's coefficient, we must first rank the observations in each sample, as noted above. In this case, the observations are already ranked; thus, if R_i and Q_i represent two vectors of ranks, Spearman's correlation coefficient, r_S, is given by the expression:

$$r_S = \frac{\sum_{i=1}^n (R_i - \overline{R})(Q_i - \overline{Q})}{\sqrt{\sum_{i=1}^n (R_i - \overline{R})^2 \sum_{i=1}^n (Q_i - \overline{Q})^2}}$$

However, for computational purposes, a more convenient expression is the following, which assumes there are no ties (if the number of ties is not too large, this simpler expression can still be used [21]):

$$r_S = 1 - \frac{6\sum_{i=1}^n (R_i - Q_i)^2}{n^3 - n}$$

The correlation between the rankings represented as **R** and **Q** in Table 1.1 above is $r_S = 0.8303$. Given that it is relatively close to 1, we conclude that the ranking **Q** is similar to ranking **R**, which represents the relevance of the documents to the given query, and is therefore a good ranking.

Now let us evaluate the alternative ranking **Z**. Spearman's correlation between this new ranking and **R** is $r_S = 0.8303$, which is exactly the same value that was obtained with **Q**. This means that both rankings, **Q** and **Z**, are equally good according to Spearman's coefficient. However, if we carefully analyze the rankings, we observe that although they are equally good *approximations* of ranking **R** as a whole, **Q** is probably more *useful* because it is more similar to **R** in the higher ranks than **Z** and not so similar in the lower ones. Assuming, as would be expected, that the higher the rank, the more probable it is that the corresponding document will actually be analyzed by the user making the query, the first ranking **Q** is clearly better than **Z**. However, as shown above, with r_S we obtain a different result because this coefficient treats all ranks equally. Thus, we need new measures of similarity between rankings that take rank importance into account.

The search for measures of weighted correlation has already been considered in a number of works in the previous years; for instance, Blest (2000), which has adapted Kendall's concordance coefficient. Blest's measure, however, is not a symmetric function of the two vectors of ranks, which makes it of little use.

In 2001 [61, 93], we have introduced the weighted rank correlation coefficient r_W whose expression is:

$$r_W = 1 - \frac{6\sum_{i=1}^n (R_i - Q_i)^2 (2n + 2 - R_i - Q_i)}{n^4 + n^3 - n^2 - n}. \tag{1.2}$$

In 2003, [28] a symmetrized version of Blest's coefficient has been presented which has later been seen to coincide with the coefficient r_W just described (see [29, 68]).

1.3 Organization of the Book

The statistical distribution of the measure of weighted correlation r_W, first for the case of independence between the two vectors of ranks and then for the general case, has been described in [63, 67], respectively. The study of the weighted measure r_W, including its asymptotic distribution, will be the subject of Chap. 2 where we will also present a simulation study and a comparison between r_W and Spearman's r_S. We will end the chapter with examples of applications of r_W.

The generalization of the coefficient r_W, which uses a linear weight function, has been given in 2007 [68] for other weight functions (see also [74]). In particular, for a quadratic weight function, we get the coefficient r_{W2},

$$r_{W2} = 1 - \frac{90 \sum_{i=1}^{n} (R_i - Q_i)^2 (2n + 2 - R_i - Q_i)^2}{n(n-1)(n+1)(2n+1)(8n+11)}, \qquad (1.3)$$

which has already been the subject of some important applications, in particular in bioinformatics [73]. In Chap. 3 a detailed exposition of this weighted correlation coefficient will be described.

In Chap. 4, we will present a new weighted Principal Component Analysis (PCA) based on this new measure r_{W2} and consider also its application to microarray data. First, a new Principal Component Analysis, introduced in [73], is presented and its robustness to outliers and noise is explained with examples. Then, a new method for selecting relevant genes in microarray data, based on this new PCA, is introduced and its comparison to other well-known methods of choosing genes in microarray data is also described. The chapter ends with the analysis of the chosen genes, for some microarray datasets, and conclusions.

In the same year of r_{W2}, 2007, a new family of conditional dependence measures and its corresponding multivariate versions, based on Spearman's rho, and related measures of tail dependence, have been introduced in [88]. These conditional dependence measures based on Spearman's rho utilize also weighting functions for specific interesting parts. In Chap. 4 of [27], the estimation of associations based also on Spearman's rho and on weighted observations is considered, together with an important area of application in finance where higher weight is given to more recent observations. This type of application where one gives different weights to more recent observations, or other regions of a time series, had also been considered in [70, 71]. There, weighted measures of association specific for time series were described and used in the context of time-dependent Principal Component Analysis and clustering of time series data.

In Chap. 5, a new weighted Principal Component Analysis, specific for time series data, will also be presented, as well as its application to a number of time series datasets. In addition, a weighted clustering specific for time series is also described in Chap. 6.

In the Appendix, some more theoretical results are presented and also tables of critical values for some of the weighted measures of correlation described in the book. In particular, the maximum value of the weighted measures of correlation is explained; the mean and variance of r_W under the null hypothesis of independence; the asymptotic normality of some nonparametric statistics which are used to prove the convergence of r_W to the Gaussian distribution; the computation of the weighted principal components in the case of having more variables than observations.

Chapter 2
The Weighted Rank Correlation Coefficient r_W

Abstract Spearman's rank correlation coefficient is not entirely suitable to measure the correlation between two rankings in some applications because it treats all ranks equally. In 2001, we have proposed a weighted rank measure of correlation that weights the distance between two ranks using a linear function of those ranks, giving more importance to higher ranks than lower ones. In this chapter, we analyze its distribution and provide a table of critical values to test whether a given value of the coefficient is significantly different from zero. We also summarize a number of applications for which the new measure is more suitable than Spearman's.

2.1 Introduction

In this chapter we analyze the statistical distribution of the weighted rank correlation coefficient r_W [61, 63, 67, 93] and provide a table of critical values to test whether a given value of the coefficient is significantly different from zero. We also summarize a number of applications for which the new measure is more suitable than Spearman's.

Rank correlation coefficients such as Spearman's [57, Chap. 9], [94] can be used to quantify the similarity between two rankings. However, Spearman's coefficient treats all ranks equally and is, therefore, not entirely suitable for applications such as the one described in the previous chapter, where different weights need to be given to different ranks.

In this chapter, we describe a measure of correlation—adapted from Spearman's rank correlation coefficient—that weighs ranks proportionally to how high they are.[1] This problem has already been considered by Blest in 2000 [10]. His measure, however, is not a symmetric function of the two vectors of ranks. The measure r_W that we have proposed in 2001 does not have this problem. In the next section, we describe rank correlation and provide an example to illustrate the need for weighted measures. In Sect. 2.3, we describe previous approaches to this problem, identifying their drawbacks, which lead us to the measure r_W described here. We also give some

---

[1]We assume that the higher rank is 1, and corresponds to the "best" element in the ranking.

© The Author(s) 2015   9
J. Pinto da Costa, *Rankings and Preferences*,
SpringerBriefs in Statistics, DOI 10.1007/978-3-662-48344-2_2

insight into its interpretation. In Sects. 2.4 and 2.5, we analyze the distribution of
the measure proposed and provide some illustrative examples. In Sect. 2.6, we dis-
cuss the applicability of the r_W measure, identify a few of its potential applications
and describe some of its limitations. Conclusions are given in Sect. 2.7. The proofs
of results used and the table of critical values of the r_W measure are given in the
Appendix.

2.2 Rank Correlation

One interesting fact about rank correlation is that, contrary to other correlation methods, it can be used not only on numerical data but on any data that can be ranked.
An example of the use of such methods is the analysis of sales data where the aim
is to assess whether there is correlation between marketing activities (i.e., visits to
clients) and the number of sales [57, Chap. 9].

Rank correlation can be applied, for instance, to the problem of evaluating rankings
of documents generated by search engines, which was introduced in the previous
chapter. As shown there, Spearman's coefficient r_S treats all ranks equally and in
that situation it should not, as the top ranks are clearly more important. Thus, we need
a measure of similarity between rankings that takes rank importance into account.
An alternative measure to r_S is Kendall's concordance coefficient [57, Chap. 9].
This coefficient is equivalent to counting the minimum number of transpositions
required to transform one ranking into the other. The most striking difference between
Spearman's and Kendall's coefficients is that the differences are squared in the former
but not in the latter. Therefore, Spearman's coefficient is more affected by larger
differences while, on the other hand, Kendall's is more affected by smaller ones.

In 2001 and 2005 [61, 63, 93], we have introduced and analyzed a weighted rank
correlation coefficient, r_W, that weighs the distance between two ranks using a linear
function of those ranks, giving more importance to higher ranks than lower ones.
This measure will be described next. We will also analyze the statistical distribution
of r_W in the case of independence between the two vectors of ranks and also for
the general case; that is, the case where we make no assumption of independence
between the two vectors of ranks. To do so, we will use the same notation and
analogous arguments of those used by Ruymgaart, Shorack and Van Zwet (1972)
in the proof of their Theorem 2.1 (see [83]). We show that r_W has a normal limit
distribution. A table of critical values for r_W will be provided in the Appendix in
order to test whether a given value of the coefficient is significantly different from
zero, and a number of applications for this new measure will also be given.

2.3 Weighted Rank Measure of Correlation

Here, we describe the construction of the weighted rank measure of correlation r_W and then use the example introduced in the previous chapter to illustrate the advantage of the new measure. As before let us denote by $R = (R_1, R_2, \ldots, R_n)$ and $Q = (Q_1, Q_2, \ldots, Q_n)$ two vectors of ranks obtained on a sample of size n.

The calculation of the distance between two ranks in Spearman's coefficient, $r_S = 1 - \frac{6 \sum_{i=1}^{n} (R_i - Q_i)^2}{n^3 - n}$, is given by:

$$D_i^2 = (R_i - Q_i)^2$$

which does not take rank importance into account. In 2000, an alternative was proposed by Soares et al. [92]: $\big((R_i - Q_i)/R_i\big)^2$. This function has several shortcomings. First, the ranking Q that will obtain the largest distance from R is not the inverted ranking, i.e., $Q_i = n - R_i + 1$, which is rather unintuitive. Second, the function is not symmetric, which means that the distance between series R and series Q can be different from the distance between Q and R. Also in 2000, an adaptation of Kendall's concordance coefficient has been proposed by Blest [10], which also addresses the same issue. However, as in the distance function proposed by Soares et al., Blest's measure is not a symmetric function of the two vectors of ranks.

Here, we use the following alternative distance measure proposed in [61, 63, 93]:

$$\begin{aligned} W_i^2 &= (R_i - Q_i)^2 \big((n - R_i + 1) + (n - Q_i + 1) \big) \\ &= D_i^2 (2n + 2 - R_i - Q_i) \end{aligned}$$

The first term of this product is D_i^2, exactly as in Spearman's method and represents the distance between R_i and Q_i. The second term represents both the importance of R_i and also the importance of Q_i.

Let us consider now again the example introduced in the previous chapter concerning the ranking of ten documents according to the relevance of each document to a particular subject. Recall that R represents the "true" ranking of the ten documents, provided by an expert, and Q and Z represent two rankings of the same ten documents provided, for instance, by two competing search engines. The sum of distances between R and Q, using this expression ($\sum_{i=1}^{n} W_i^2$), is 278 and the sum of distances between R and Z is 436 (Table 2.1). This means that the distance between R and Z is larger, a conclusion that is consistent with the intuitive analysis of the usefulness of suggested rankings in the previous section. In fact, given that ranking R is more similar to ranking Q in the most important ranks, the first ones, we expect the difference between rankings R and Q to be smaller, which is the case. As for Spearman's coefficient both distances, between rankings R and Q and rankings R and Z are the same, which is rather unintuitive.

Now, in order to construct a correlation coefficient based on this new distance, we will follow a common strategy, which consists in looking for an affine function of

Table 2.1 Application of the new distance measure to the example of rankings of documents

Document	R	Q			Z		
i	R_i	Q_i	D_i^2	W_i^2	Z_i	D_i^2	W_i^2
D1	1	2	1	19	3	4	72
D2	2	1	1	19	5	9	135
D3	3	4	1	15	2	1	17
D4	4	6	4	48	1	9	153
D5	5	5	0	0	6	1	11
D6	6	3	9	117	4	4	48
D7	7	8	1	7	7	0	0
D8	8	9	1	5	8	0	0
D9	9	10	1	3	9	0	0
D10	10	7	9	45	10	0	0
Sum				278			436

the distance between the two rankings, an expression of the form $A + B \sum_1^n W_i^2$. The idea is to find which two constants A and B make this expression to take values in $[-1, 1]$, as is usual with correlation coefficients; 1 when they are the same ($R_i = Q_i$) and -1 when the rankings are inverted ($R_i = n + 1 - Q_i$). In the first case, we have that $\sum_1^n W_i^2 = 0$ and so A must be 1. In the second case, as is shown in Appendix A.1, the maximum value of the weighted distance $\sum_1^n W_i^2$ between two rankings is $(n^4 + n^3 - n^2 - n)/3$ and is obtained when the rankings are inverted, that is, $Q_i = n + 1 - R_i$. Using this expression for the maximum value of the weighted distance, we obtain therefore that $A + B \cdot (n^4 + n^3 - n^2 - n)/3 = -1$. Using these two conditions for the two constants A and B, the weighted rank measure of correlation, $r_W = A + B \sum_1^n W_i^2$, becomes, after some simplifications:

$$r_W = 1 - \frac{6 \sum_{i=1}^n (R_i - Q_i)^2 \big((n - R_i + 1) + (n - Q_i + 1) \big)}{n^4 + n^3 - n^2 - n} \qquad (2.1)$$

In the example of Table 2.1 concerning the ranking of documents, the r_W value for R and Q is 0.8468. As expected, this is higher than the r_W value for R and Z, which is 0.7598.

As stated earlier, rank correlation coefficients measure the monotonicity between two series of matched values. We have just described the weighted r_W measure of correlation, adapted from Spearman's r_S, that takes rank importance into account, unlike the latter. That is, correlation will be more affected by points that are ranked higher in the series than others. Next we analyze the statistical distribution of this measure, starting with the case of independence between the two vectors of ranks. We also analyze the differences between Spearman's r_S and the weighted measure r_W.

2.4 Properties of the Distribution of r_W Under the Null Hypothesis of Independence

In this section, we will study the distribution of r_W under the null hypothesis of independence between the two vectors of rankings. We start by briefly describing some results from linear rank statistics, which will be used next to determine the expected value and the variance of r_W. We provide evidence to suggest that, under the null hypothesis, the standardized value of r_W follows the Gaussian distribution; that is,

$$(r_W - E(r_W))/\sqrt{\text{var}(r_W)} \overset{d}{\approx} N(0, 1)$$

As above, let us denote by $\boldsymbol{R} = (R_1, \ldots, R_n)$ the first vector of ranks and by $\boldsymbol{Q} = (Q_1, \ldots, Q_n)$ the second vector of ranks. That is, $\boldsymbol{R}$ and $\boldsymbol{Q}$ assume only values in the set $\mathscr{R}$ of all the $n!$ permutations of the integers $(1, \ldots, n)$. Under the null hypothesis,

$$H_0 : \boldsymbol{R} \text{ and } \boldsymbol{Q} \text{ are independent,}$$

the two rank vectors are both uniformly distributed over $\mathscr{R}$. This implies that the distribution of

$$r_W = 1 - \frac{6 \sum_{i=1}^{n} (R_i - Q_i)^2 (2(n+1) - R_i - Q_i)}{n(n^3 + n^2 - n - 1)}$$

is the same as the distribution of

$$1 - \frac{6 \sum_{i=1}^{n} (i - R_i^*)^2 (2(n+1) - i - R_i^*)}{n(n^3 + n^2 - n - 1)}$$

where $\boldsymbol{R}^* = (R_1^*, \ldots, R_n^*)$ is a random vector taken uniformly from the set $\mathscr{R}$.

2.4.1 Linear Rank Statistics

A statistic of the form

$$S = \sum_{i=1}^{n} c(i)a(R_i^*) \tag{2.2}$$

is called a linear rank statistic [78, Chap. 8]. The constants $a(1), \ldots, a(n)$ are called the scores and $c(1), \ldots, c(n)$ the regression constants. In [78, Chap. 8] it is shown that, under H_0,

(i) $\Pr(R_i^* = r) = \frac{1}{n}, r = 1, \ldots, n$

(ii) if $i \neq j$ then $\Pr(R_i^* = r, R_j^* = s) = \begin{cases} \frac{1}{n(n-1)} & r \neq s = 1, \ldots, n; \\ 0 & \text{otherwise} \end{cases}$ (2.3)

(iii) $E(S) = n\bar{c}\,\bar{a}$

(iv) $\text{var}(S) = (n-1)s_c^2 s_a^2,$

where $\bar{a}$ and $\bar{c}$ represent the average values of the scores and regression constants, respectively. Similarly, s_a^2 and s_c^2 represent their variances.

We will now find the two first moments of the weighted rank correlation coefficient r_W under the hypothesis of independence between the two vectors of ranks. In particular, its expected value has the desirable property of being equal to zero under independence, which is a common result for correlation coefficients.

Theorem 1 *Under the hypothesis of independence between two vectors of ranks,*

$$E(r_W) = 0 \text{ and } \text{var}(r_W) = \frac{31n^2 + 60n + 26}{30(n^3 + n^2 - n - 1)}$$

The proof is given in Appendix A.3.

2.4.2 Exact and Asymptotic Distribution of r_W Under the Null Hypothesis of Independence

We will now investigate the asymptotic distribution of $(r_W - E(r_W))/\sqrt{\text{var}(r_W)}$, under the null hypothesis of independence between the two vectors of ranks. Let

$$S_n^{(11)} = \sum_{i=1}^{n} iR_i^*, \qquad S_n^{(12)} = \sum_{i=1}^{n} iR_i^{*2}, \qquad S_n^{(21)} = \sum_{i=1}^{n} i^2 R_i^*$$

Then, as shown in the Appendix,

$$r_W = \frac{1}{n(n^3 + n^2 - n - 1)} \left(24(n+1)\left(S_n^{(11)} - E\left(S_n^{(11)} \right) \right) \right.$$
$$\left. -6\left(S_n^{(12)} - E(S_n^{(12)}) \right) - 6\left(S_n^{(21)} - E(S_n^{(21)}) \right) \right)$$

To standardize r_W, we divide by the square root of its variance ($E(r_W) = 0$ under the null hypothesis). We start by defining the three constants,

$$a_n^{(11)} = \frac{2\sqrt{30}n(n+1)^2\sqrt{n-1}}{n\sqrt{31n^2 + 60n + 26}\sqrt{n^3 + n^2 - n - 1}},$$

$$a_n^{(12)} = \frac{-6\sqrt{30}n(n+1)\frac{\sqrt{16n^3 + 14n^2 - 19n - 11}}{2160}}{n\sqrt{31n^2 + 60n + 26}\sqrt{n^3 + n^2 - n - 1}}$$

$$a_n^{(21)} = \frac{-6\sqrt{30}n(n+1)\frac{\sqrt{16n^3+14n^2-19n-11}}{2160}}{n\sqrt{31n^2+60n+26}\sqrt{n^3+n^2-n-1}}$$

Then,

$$\frac{r_W}{\sqrt{\text{var}(r_W)}} = a_n^{(11)}\frac{S_n^{(11)} - \mu_n^{(11)}}{\sigma_n^{(11)}} + a_n^{(12)}\frac{S_n^{(12)} - \mu_n^{(12)}}{\sigma_n^{(12)}} + a_n^{(21)}\frac{S_n^{(21)} - \mu_n^{(21)}}{\sigma_n^{(21)}}$$

where

$$\mu_n^{(k\ell)} = \text{E}(S_n^{(k\ell)}) \quad \text{and} \quad \sigma_n^{(k\ell)} = \sqrt{\text{var}(S_n^{(k\ell)})}$$

In [78, Chap. 8] it is shown that as $n \longrightarrow \infty$ the following statistic converges in distribution to the Gaussian:

$$\frac{S_n^{(k\ell)} - \mu_n^{(k\ell)}}{\sigma_n^{(k\ell)}} \xrightarrow{d} N(0,1)$$

On the other hand, as $n \longrightarrow \infty$,

$$a_n^{(11)} \longrightarrow a^{(11)} = 2\sqrt{\frac{30}{31}}, \quad a_n^{(12)} \longrightarrow a^{(12)} = -\frac{1}{90}\sqrt{\frac{30}{31}} \quad \text{and} \quad a_n^{(21)} \longrightarrow a^{(21)} = a^{(12)}$$

Therefore [8, p. 288],

$$a_n^{(k\ell)}\frac{S_n^{(k\ell)} - \mu_n^{(k\ell)}}{\sigma_n^{(k\ell)}} \xrightarrow{d} a^{(k\ell)}Z$$

where Z stands for the standard normal distribution. So, the standardized r_W is the sum of three statistics that are asymptotically normal. However, these three statistics are not independent and so we cannot conclude directly that their sum is asymptotically normal.

In order to verify the asymptotic distribution of r_W, we have started by computing some theoretical and empirical distributions in the next section, and compared it with the normal curve.

2.4.3 Simulations

We have calculated the exact distribution of r_W for n up to 14. Due to computational limitations, for larger values of n, we estimated the distribution based on a random sample of one million permutations. For $n = 14$, we observe that there is a small difference between the exact and estimated values for the most important quantiles (Table 2.2). Note that we have decided not to interpolate the critical values because it is a discrete distribution. Instead, we used a common strategy of finding the quantiles

Table 2.2 Difference between the exact and estimated quantiles for $n = 14$

Quantile (%)	0.5	1	2.5	5	95	97.5	99	99.5
Difference	0.0052	0.0042	0.0021	0.0000	0.0010	0.0010	0.0010	0.0010

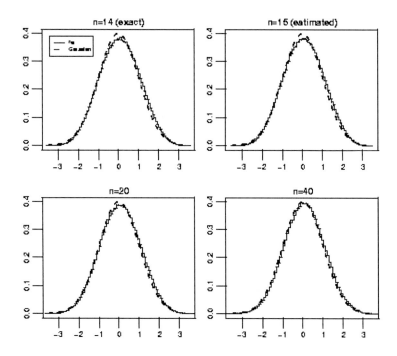

Fig. 2.1 Exact distribution for $n = 14$ and estimated distribution for $n = 15, 20$ and 40, together with the Standard Normal curve

of a discrete distribution but with a slight change. With a discrete distribution, all the values in a given interval satisfy the definition of quantile of order p. This might bring a difficulty in choosing the quantile especially for small n. Therefore, for each confidence level α_i, we have multiplied it by the total number of permutations, $n!$. If the result is not an integer, we use the next lower/higher integer for small/large confidence levels, respectively. Finally, we picked the corresponding order statistic.

In Fig. 2.1, we plot the distribution for $n = 14$ and $n = 15$, respectively, the last exact and the first estimated distributions. The graphs indicate that the sample size is adequate. In the same figure, we also plot the estimated distributions for $n = 20$ and 40, respectively. In all graphs, the values of r_W have been standardized and we plot the normal curve for comparison.

The empirical distribution of r_W does not lie symmetrically about zero. This is because the distribution of the values of our statistic is not symmetric; it is a little skewed. This does not strike us as a problem, since we think there is no reason for a

Fig. 2.2 Difference between the estimated quantiles of r_W and the quantiles of the Standard Normal

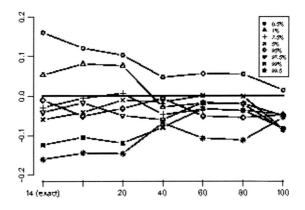

measure of correlation to be necessarily symmetric. The measure r_W was constructed so that the first ranks are more important than the other ranks and this influences its symmetry. Unlike Blest's measure, our statistic treats both rankings similarly; that is, $r_W(\mathbf{R},\mathbf{Q}) = r_W(\mathbf{Q},\mathbf{R})$. However, this does not mean that the distribution of its values, which lie in the interval $(-1, 1)$, is symmetric. In fact it is not. For instance, for $n = 3$, the values of the statistic are $-1, -0.5, -0.5, 0.375, 0.625$, and 1; these values have mean zero, but are not symmetric about zero. For the same reason, the percentiles are also not symmetric about zero (e.g., the 5 % and 95 % percentiles for $n = 5$, which are given in Table A.1 (Appendix), are not the same in absolute value).

We have calculated the difference between the quantiles for the standardized r_W and the standard normal for a few values of n and observed that the differences are small (Fig. 2.2). For $n > 40$, we have observed that these differences are always smaller than 0.1. This means that the differences between the nonstandardized r_W and the approximation given by the normal distribution is smaller than $0.1\sqrt{\mathrm{var}(r_W)}$. For instance, for $n = 51$, the difference between r_W and the approximation given by the normal curve is smaller than 0.003.

2.4.4 Comparison Between r_W and r_S

In the last subsections, we have presented an adaptation of Spearman's rank correlation coefficient, which assigns more importance to higher ranks. Here we start with a comparison of the weighted measure r_W with Spearman's coefficient r_S to point out the differences and describe the conditions under which the new coefficient should be used.

Despite the similarities between the two measures r_W and r_S, they may yield quite different values when applied to the same pair of series. We illustrate these differences using a few examples.

We start by measuring the correlation between rankings $\mathbf{R}$ and $\mathbf{Q}$. The former is defined as $\mathbf{R} = (1, 2, \dots, n - 1, n)$, where n is the number of elements in the ranking. Ranking Q is obtained from R by swapping the elements $(1, \ldots, p)$ and $(q - p + 1, \ldots, q)$, after inverting the order in each of them:

$$R = \quad (\boxed{1, \ldots, p}, \; p+1, \ldots, q-p, \; \boxed{q-p+1, \ldots, q}, \; q+1, \ldots, n)$$

$$Q = (\boxed{q, \ldots, q-p+1}, \; p+1, \ldots, q-p, \; \boxed{p, \ldots, 1}, \qquad q+1, \ldots, n).$$

We plot in Fig. 2.3 the value of $r_W(R,Q) - r_S(R,Q)$ for a few values of n, p, and q. Note that although some of the differences are already quite large, achieving values close to 0.15, it is possible to obtain even larger differences. Furthermore, if both p and q are represented as proportions of n, the differences are independent of the size of the ranking (in the examples the differences decrease with the size of the ranking, n, because we have used values of p which represent smaller proportions).

Having proved that the two rank correlation coefficients, r_W adn r_S, can give quite different results, it is of importance now to decide when to use r_W. The new measure should be used instead of Spearman's coefficient in applications for which it is known that the importance of concordance between the series decreases with the ranks. In other words, assuming that $f(i)$ is a function that represents the importance of rank i, r_W should be used rather than r_S if:

$$i < j \Rightarrow f(i) > f(j). \tag{2.4}$$

Note that we assume that 1 is the highest rank and n is the lowest one, where n is the number of elements in the series. Again, let us illustrate with some more examples. We measure the difference between the weighted correlation of a ranking R and each of two rankings Q and Z, i.e., $r_W(R, Q) - r_W(R, Z)$. As before, $R = (1, 2, \ldots, n-1, n)$, where n is the number of elements. Ranking Q is obtained from R by swapping the elements $(1, \ldots, p)$ and $(q + 1, \ldots, q + p)$:

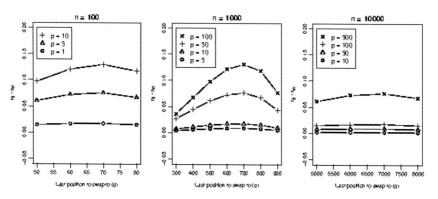

Fig. 2.3 Difference between Spearman's coefficient (r_S) and the new weighted measure of correlation (r_W) on a few illustrative examples

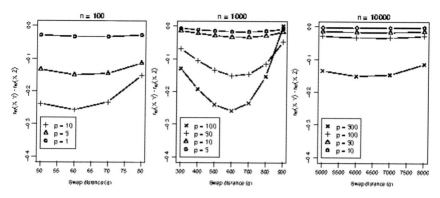

Fig. 2.4 Difference between two weighted rank correlation values, $r_W(\mathbf{R}, \mathbf{Q})$ and $r_W(\mathbf{R}, \mathbf{Z})$, where $\mathbf{Q}$ and $\mathbf{Z}$ are obtained by applying a symmetric procedure to $\mathbf{R}$, for a few illustrative examples of different parameters of the procedure

$$\mathbf{R} = (\,\boxed{1, \ldots, p}\,, \; p+1, \ldots, q, \; \boxed{q+1, \ldots, q+p}\,, \; q+p+1, \ldots, n)$$

$$\mathbf{Q} = (\,\boxed{q+1, \ldots, q+p}\,, \; p+1, \ldots, q, \; \boxed{1, \ldots, p}\,, \qquad q+p+1, \ldots, n).$$

Ranking $\mathbf{Z}$ is obtained from $\mathbf{R}$ using a symmetric procedure to the one used to generate $\mathbf{Q}$. We swap the elements $(n-p+1, \ldots, n)$ and $(n-q-p+1, \ldots, n-q)$:

$$\mathbf{R} = (1, \ldots, n-q-p, \; \boxed{n-q-p+1, \ldots, n-q}\,,$$
$$n-q+1, \ldots, n-p, \; \boxed{n-p+1, \ldots, n}\,)$$

$$\mathbf{Z} = (1, \ldots, n-q-p, \; \boxed{n-p+1, \ldots, n}\,,$$
$$n-q+1, \ldots, n-p, \; \boxed{n-q-p+1, \ldots, n-q}\,)$$

According to the assumption above (2.4), the concordance between $\mathbf{R}$ and $\mathbf{Z}$ is clearly much higher than between $\mathbf{R}$ and $\mathbf{Q}$. However, the value of r_S is the same in both cases. The difference between the values of the weighted measure in the two cases is illustrated in Fig. 2.4 for a few values of n, p, and q.

Note that we have made a very weak assumption, (2.4), namely that the higher the rank, the higher its importance. This enables us to consider a wide range of applications, a few of which are enumerated in Sect. 2.6. However, in some applications it is possible to make stronger assumptions. For instance, it may be known that only the top 1, 5, or 10 alternatives in the ranking will be considered. In these cases, it may be more suitable to use more specific measures that only take those ranks into consideration and ignore all the others. Other weighted measures of correlation will be given in later chapters.

Our main claim is that the weighted measure r_W is more appropriate than traditional rank correlation coefficients for a wide range of applications where higher ranks are more important than lower ones. Although r_W gives more importance to higher ranks, it still takes the whole ranking into account rather than simply assuming that some ranks matter and others do not. Therefore, it may be used as a general measure of similarity between two rankings. By treating rankings as a whole, generality is gained (i.e., it may be applied to a wide range of ranking problems) at the cost of the ability to capture specificities of individual problems (e.g., only the top-5 ranks are considered). Therefore, we do not claim that it should replace problem-specific measures. We believe that it may be more useful as a complement to those measures, assessing the general concordance between rankings, while other measures may provide a more specific assessment.

2.5 The Asymptotic Distribution of r_W for the General Case

In the last section we have seen that, in the case of independence between two rankings, the weighted measure of correlation r_W seems to converge to the Gaussian distribution, according to the simulations realized. Now we make no independence assumptions; that is, we study the asymptotic distribution of r_W for the general case and we give the formal proof that r_W converges to the normal distribution (see also [67]). This section is rather technical and can be skipped at a first reading. First,

$$r_W = 1 - \frac{6\sum_{i=1}^{n}(R_i - Q_i)^2(2n + 2 - R_i - Q_i)}{n^4 + n^3 - n^2 - n}$$

$$= 1 - \frac{6}{n}\sum_{i=1}^{n}\left(\frac{R_i}{n+1} - \frac{Q_i}{n+1}\right)^2\left(\frac{2n + 2 - R_i - Q_i}{n - 1}\right)$$

Therefore, the asymptotic behavior of r_W is the same as the one of $1 - 6W_n$, where

$$W_n = \frac{1}{n}\sum_{i=1}^{n}\left(\frac{R_i}{n+1} - \frac{Q_i}{n+1}\right)^2\left(2 - \frac{R_i}{n+1} - \frac{Q_i}{n+1}\right).$$

W_n is a statistic of the type $\frac{1}{n}\sum_{i=1}^{n}a_n(R_i, Q_i)$, where $a_n(i, j)$ is a real number for $i, j = 1, 2, \ldots, n$.

If we define $J(s, t) = (s - t)^2(2 - s - t), 0 \leq s, t \leq 1$, then $J(s, t)$ is a limit of the score function,

$$J_n(s, t) = a_n(i, j) = J\left(\frac{i}{n+1}, \frac{j}{n+1}\right), \tag{2.5}$$

for i and j such that $\frac{i-1}{n} < s \le \frac{i}{n}$ and $\frac{j-1}{n} < t \le \frac{j}{n}$. Hence, W_n can be written as (see [7]),

$$W_n = \int \int J_n(F_n, G_n) dH_n, \tag{2.6}$$

where F_n and G_n are the empirical marginal distribution functions of F and G, respectively; H_n is the bivariate empirical distribution function of H. Now, let us define the population moment $\mu = \int \int J(F, G) dH$. By analogy to r_W, we define the population weighted rank correlation coefficient between two variables X and Y to be,

$$\rho_W(X, Y) = 1 - 6\mu$$

$$= 1 - 6 \int \int (F(x) - G(y))^2 (2 - F(x) - G(y)) dH(x, y),$$

or, by using copulas [58]

$$\rho_W(X, Y) = 1 - 6 \int_{[0,1]^2} (u - v)^2 (2 - u - v) dc(u, v),$$

where the copula $c(u, v) = P(F(X) \le u, G(y) \le v), 0 \le u, v \le 1$.

Next, we present the conclusion that r_W is asymptotically Gaussian distributed.

Theorem 2.1 *r_W is an asymptotic normal and consistent (ANC) estimator of ρ_W*

Proof We want to prove that r_W is an asymptotic normal and consistent (ANC) estimator of ρ_W; first,

$$\sqrt{n}(r_W - \rho_W) = -6\sqrt{n}(W_n - \mu) = -6\sqrt{n}\left[\int \int J_n(F_n, G_n) dH_n - \mu \right].$$

We start by considering the empirical processes $U_n(F) = \sqrt{n}(F_n - F)$, $V_n(G) = \sqrt{n}(G_n - G)$, $U_n^*(F) = \sqrt{n}(F_n^* - F)$, $V_n^*(G) = \sqrt{n}(G_n^* - G)$, where $F_n^* = \left[\frac{n}{n+1} F_n \right]$ and $G_n^* = \left[\frac{n}{n+1} G_n \right]$. Let now $\bar{\Delta}_n = [X_{1n}, X_{nn}] \times [Y_{1n}, Y_{nn}]$ where X_{in} and Y_{in} denote the ith order statistics and $B_{0n}^* = \sqrt{n} \int \int \left[J_n(F_n, G_n) - J(F_n^*, G_n^*) \right] dH_n$.

We will now prove that $J_n(F_n, G_n) = J(F_n^*, G_n^*)$ and so $B_{0n}^* = 0$ for all n. In fact, the function F_n, for instance, is a step function and so there is always an $i \in \{0, 1, \ldots, n\}$ such that $F_n = \frac{i}{n}$; similarly for G_n. This means that by (2.5) $J_n(F_n, G_n) = J\left(\frac{i}{n+1}, \frac{j}{n+1} \right)$ for some i and j. Now, by the definition above, $\frac{i}{n+1} = F_n^*$ and $\frac{j}{n+1} = G_n^*$. So, $B_{0n}^* = 0$ for all n.

Because $B_{0n}^* = 0$ for all n, then an assumption similar to 2.3(b) in [83] (see Appendix A.5) is satisfied, that is, $B_{0n}^* \to_p 0$. We will now use the same argument of these authors, adapting it to our situation because our score function $a_n(i, j)$ is bivariate and the score functions used in [83], $a_n(i)$ and $b_n(i)$ have just one variable (see Appendix A.5). Nevertheless, the adaption follows from the same steps of their proof. The asymptotic convergence of r_W to the normal distribution may be uniform over a class of distribution functions. However, in this work, we are not interested in proving uniform convergence, but only convergence for a single distribution.

Now we can write,

$$\sqrt{n}(W_n - \mu) = \sum_{i=1}^{3} A_{in} + B_{0n}^* + B_{1n}^*,$$

where

$$A_{1n} = \sqrt{n} \int \int J(F, G)d(H_n - H), \ A_{2n} = \int \int U_n(F)\frac{\partial J}{\partial s}(F, G)dH,$$
$$A_{3n} = \int \int V_n(G)\frac{\partial J}{\partial t}(F, G)dH, \ B_{0n}^* \text{ is defined above; and}$$
$$B_{1n}^* = \sqrt{n} \int \int \left[J(F_n^*, G_n^*) - J(F, G)\right] dH_n - A_{2n} - A_{3n}.$$

2.5.1 $\sum_{i=1}^{3} A_{in}$ is Asymptotically Normal Distributed

As in [83], we can prove the asymptotic normality of A_{1n}, A_{2n}, and A_{3n} based on the fact that J is a continuous function and its partial derivatives are continuous and bounded on $(0, 1)^2$.

Let us start by noting that $A_{1n} = \frac{1}{\sqrt{n}} \sum_{i=1}^{n} A_{1in}$ where $A_{1in} = J(F(X_i), G(Y_i)) - \mu$. In fact,

$$A_{1n} = \sqrt{n} \int \int J(F, G)d(H_n - H) = \sqrt{n} \left(\int \int J(F, G)dH_n - \int \int J(F, G)dH \right)$$

Now, as in Eq. 2.6 we get,

$$A_{1n} = \frac{\sqrt{n}}{n} \sum_{i=1}^{n} (J(F(X_i), G(Y_i)) - \mu)$$

$$= \frac{1}{\sqrt{n}} \sum_{i=1}^{n} (J(F(X_i), G(Y_i)) - \mu).$$

The random variables A_{1in} are independent and identically distributed (i.i.d.) with mean zero. If we choose $\delta = \frac{1}{4}$, $D = p_0 = q_0 = 2$, $r(u) = \frac{1}{u(1-u)}$ then we have an assumption similar to Assumption 2.1 in the statement of Theorem 2.1 in [83] (See Appendix A), that is, $J(F, G) \leq D(r(F))^a (r(G))^b$ with $a = \frac{\delta - \frac{1}{2}}{p_0} = -\frac{1}{8}$ and $b = \frac{\delta - \frac{1}{2}}{q_0} = -\frac{1}{8}$; $\frac{\partial J}{\partial s}(F, G) \leq D(r(F))^{a+1} (r(G))^b$ with $a = \frac{\delta - \frac{1}{2}}{p_1} = -\frac{1}{8}$ and

$b = \frac{\delta - \frac{1}{2}}{q1} = -\frac{1}{8}$ and $\frac{\partial J}{\partial t}(F, G) \leq D(r(F))^b(r(G))^{a+1}$ with $a = \frac{\delta - \frac{1}{2}}{p2} = -\frac{1}{8}$ and

$b = \frac{\delta - \frac{1}{2}}{q2} = -\frac{1}{8}$.

Taking this assumption into account and by application of Hölder's inequality,

$$\int\int |\phi(F)\psi(G)| \, dH \leq \left[\int |\phi|^{p_0} \, dI\right]^{\frac{1}{p_0}} \left[\int |\psi|^{q_0} \, dI\right]^{\frac{1}{q_0}},$$

$$\forall p_0 > 0, q_o > 0 : \frac{1}{p_0} + \frac{1}{q_0} = 1;$$

where ϕ and ψ are functions on $(0, 1)$, dI denotes Lebesgue measure restricted to the unit interval, we note that A_{1in} has a finite absolute moment of order $2 + \delta_0$ for some $\delta_0 > 0$ (see Appendix A.6).

Let us consider now A_{2n}. As $U_n(F) = \frac{1}{\sqrt{n}} \sum_{i=1}^{n}(I(X_i \leq x) - F)$ we can write $A_{2n} = \frac{1}{\sqrt{n}} \sum_{i=1}^{n} A_{2in}$, where $A_{2in} = \int\int (I(X_i \leq x) - F)\frac{\partial J}{\partial s}(F, G)dH$ are i.i.d with mean zero. If we choose $\delta = \frac{1}{4}$, $D = p_1 = q_1 = 2$, $r(u) = \frac{1}{u(1-u)}$ then an assumption similar to 2.1 in [83] is satisfied. Again, by applying Hölder's inequality and similarly to A_{1in}, it follows that A_{2in} has a finite absolute moment of order $2 + \delta_1$ for some $\delta_1 > 0$.

Let us consider now A_{3n}. As $V_n(G) = \frac{1}{\sqrt{n}} \sum_{i=1}^{n}(I(Y_i \leq y) - G)$ we can write $A_{3n} = \frac{1}{\sqrt{n}} \sum_{i=1}^{n} A_{3in}$ where $A_{3in} = \int\int (I(Y_i \leq y) - G)\frac{\partial J}{\partial t}(F, G)dH$ are i.i.d with mean zero. If we choose $\delta = \frac{1}{4}$, $D = p_2 = q_2 = 2$, $r(u) = \frac{1}{u(1-u)}$ then an assumption similar to assumption 2.1 in [83], is satisfied. By application of Hölder's inequality and similarly to A_{1in}, it follows that A_{3in} has a finite absolute moment of order $2 + \delta_2$ for some $\delta_2 > 0$.

From the above conclusions: $A_{1n} = \frac{1}{\sqrt{n}} \sum_{i=1}^{n} A_{1in}$ where A_{1in} are i.i.d. with mean zero; $A_{2n} = \frac{1}{\sqrt{n}} \sum_{i=1}^{n} A_{2in}$ where A_{2in} are i.i.d with mean zero; $A_{3n} = \frac{1}{\sqrt{n}} \sum_{i=1}^{n} A_{3in}$ where A_{3in} are i.i.d with mean zero and because $A_{1in}, A_{2in}, A_{3in}$ have a finite absolute moment of order larger than 2, we get $\sum_{i=1}^{3} A_{in} \to_d N(0, \sigma^2)$ as $n \to \infty$. The expression for the variance corresponds to Eq. 3.10 in [83] and is given by

$$\sigma^2 = Var\left[J(F(X), G(Y)) + \int\int (I(X \leq x) - F)\frac{\partial J}{\partial s}(F(x), G(y))dH(x, y)\right.$$

$$\left. + \int\int (I(Y \leq y) - G)\frac{\partial J}{\partial t}(F(x), G(y))dH(x, y)\right].$$

2.5.2 B_{1n}^* is Asymptotically Negligible

We have already seen that an assumption similar to 2.3(b) in [83] is satisfied. If we consider the mean value theorem (see [84]),

$$\sqrt{n}J(F_n^*, G_n^*) = \sqrt{n}J(F, G) + U_n^*(F)\frac{\partial J}{\partial s}(\phi_n^*, \psi_n^*) + V_n^*(G)\frac{\partial J}{\partial t}(\phi_n^*, \psi_n^*)$$

for all (x, y) in $\bar{\Delta}_n$ with $\phi_n^* = F + \alpha_3(F_n^* - F)$ and $\psi_n^* = G + \alpha_4(G_n^* - G)$, where α_3 and α_4 are numbers between 0 and 1, then B_{1n}^* can be decomposed as a sum of seven terms ($\sum_{i=1}^5 B_{\gamma in}^* + B_{6n}^* + C_n^*$) which are all asymptotically negligible by the same arguments used in Sects. 5 and 6 of Ruymgaart et al. [83].

2.5.3 r_W is Asymptotically Normal Distributed

We have thus that $\sqrt{n}(W_n - \mu) \to N(0, \sigma^2)$ in distribution and it is immediate that r_W is an asymptotic normal and consistent (ANC) estimator of ρ_W: $\sqrt{n}(r_W - \rho_W) \to N(0, 36\sigma^2)$.

2.6 Examples of Application of r_W

The motivation underlying this work applies to a broad range of applications involving rankings of alternatives representing the preferences stated by humans or recommendations provided by decision support systems.

A general application is the evaluation of methods to predict rankings. The evaluation of these methods consists of comparing the ranking R of a set of n objects generated by a ranking prediction method for a given situation with the target ranking Q of the same set of objects on the same situation. A few examples of ranking prediction applications are recommendation of data analysis tools, stock trading support, information retrieval, recommender systems and user preferences, which will be discussed in more detail next.

The recommendation of data analysis tools is an important problem in knowledge discovery in databases (KDD) or data mining. Due to its interactive and iterative nature, an important part of the KDD process is often spent trying different preprocessing methods (e.g., discretization of numeric attributes) and learning algorithms (e.g., decision trees or support vector machines), and tuning their parameters [12].

One of the first applications that have been considered and that was indeed one of the motivations to develop weighted correlation coefficients comes from the field of machine learning; more precisely, meta-learning: given a certain number of algorithms to perform a given task, one would like to rank those algorithms from 1, the most adequate, to n, the worst. Then, given a certain method to recommend the algorithms, the weighted correlation coefficient r_W is used to evaluate the method. This is not a usual machine learning problem. Traditionally, the supervised learning approach to problems where each example can be a member of one set of n possible classes is *classification*. That is, a set of prelabelled examples is used to induce a model that selects a single one of those classes as the prediction for a new example. In this approach, a lot of information that can be useful in some situations is lost, because none but the "best" class is kept.

In the problem of selecting the best algorithm for a given task [91], for instance, a classification approach would provide one suggestion of an algorithm. We thus would know that the suggested algorithm is expected to be the best but no information about the other candidates algorithms is given. In this case, a ranking of the alternative algorithms (i.e., classes) provides complete information about the expected relative performance of all candidates and enables a more flexible decision process. The user may simply decide to run the algorithm ranked highest but he or she may also, if enough time or computational resources are available, decide to try the first few alternatives. An expert user might even have reasons to ignore the first recommendation, opting, for instance, to use the recommendation in the second rank.

As our example shows, rankings are particularly important for meta-learning, i.e., algorithm selection using past performance information [44, 56, 91]. Other areas where it may be advantageous to use a ranking approach, rather than the usual supervised classification, are medicine (e.g., diagnosis of an illness or choice of an adequate test or treatment) and control systems (e.g., choice of the correct action to carry out). Two areas where rankings are already widely used are information retrieval [53] and recommender systems [87].

Given that ranking is a learning task different from existing ones, like classification, regression, or clustering, it requires different evaluation procedures. That is in the evaluation process of ranking that the weighted correlation coefficient will be used and indeed this application was one of the driving forces for the development of weighted correlation coefficients. In [61, 93], an evaluation framework has been developed that consists of comparing the ranking suggested by the ranking method, called the *recommended ranking*, with the true ranking, called the *ideal ranking* [11]. The two rankings can be compared by using, for instance, a rank correlation coefficient. Nevertheless, as is obvious in this application, the top ranks are the most important; the user will try one, two, or maybe three of the top recommended ranks, but will probably have no time or resources to try all of the n orderings. Therefore it is very important that the *recommended ranking* is similar to the *ideal ranking* in the top ranks and it is not so important that the two rankings are similar in the last positions. The first idea to compare the two rankings was by means of the Spearman correlation coefficient; nevertheless, as this coefficient gives the same importance (weight) to all of the ranks, the results were not good. This motivated thus the development of the correlation coefficient r_W described above, that appeared for the first time in [61, 93], and was later developed in [63, 67].

The evaluation of stock trading support systems is also a potential application of the weighted rank measure of correlation. This problem has traditionally been tackled as a regression (i.e., predict the value of an individual stock) or as a supervised classification problem (i.e., predict whether to buy, keep or sell a stock). However, what investors want is, in fact, to have a grading of the stocks in question, such that they can make a decision concerning which ones to invest in [35]. Such a grading can be represented as a ranking. The accuracy of a system that predicts the ranking of a set of stocks could be evaluated by measuring the correlation between the predicted ranking to the true ranking of the stocks. To maximize profit, the stocks ranked higher are more important than the ones with lower ranks. Therefore, weighted measures would be more suitable to evaluate such a system than traditional ones.

Two problems that are usually handled as ranking tasks are information retrieval [4] and recommender systems [14]. Evaluation strategies in these areas, usually handle the uncertainty concerning how many alternatives will actually be tried out by the user, by simulating a number of different Top-N scenarios, i.e., by assuming that the user will select the N higher ranked alternatives for different values of N (e.g., 1, 5, 10, etc.). The corresponding results are either presented to the user (possibly represented in a chart) or summarized into one value. However, although the problems that motivated this work are equally relevant in the evaluation of information retrieval systems [4], correlation-based evaluation is not very common, except in the problem of database selection, where Spearman's coefficient has been used [18]. This is true despite the most commonly used evaluation measures are based on relevance assessment, which is an arguable approach [33]. Surprisingly, rank importance is rarely taken into account [40]. Similar remarks can also be made concerning recommender systems [14].

An example which also involves both rankings representing human preferences and generated by models, is the work of [9]. This work investigates methods to infer user preferences concerning health profiles. Evaluation is performed by comparing the predicted rankings to explicitly stated rankings. The authors have used Spearman's r_S to assess ranking similarity. However, it is common knowledge that when stating their preference as rankings, humans rank the most preferred alternatives, i.e., the ones ranked at the top, more accurately than the others. Therefore, the weighted measure r_W or other would be more appropriate than the traditional one.

Many other examples could be given where weighted correlation makes sense, as for instance in bioinformatics. In Chap. 4 we describe an application of weighted correlation in gene expression data where it is clear that the higher absolute expression values in microarray data are more important. Also, weighted correlation is not only important in the application per se, but also because it allowed the development of a new method of weighted Principal Component Analysis.

2.7 Conclusions About r_W

In this chapter, we describe a new rank measure of correlation r_W. It is applicable to problems where the level of correlation between two series of rankings is affected by the importance of each rank. We compare the new measure with Spearman's rank correlation coefficient and show that the weighted measure is clearly more suitable for such problems.

In r_W, we have used a linear rank weighting function to assign more importance to higher ranks (the first ranks). Although r_W is more suitable than Spearman's r_S for the type of applications we are concerned with, like those just described, the linear function may not be the best one in all of them. In the next chapter, we will analyze whether other weighting functions can be more adequate for specific situations. In information retrieval and recommender systems, for instance, the exponential weight function has been used in problem-specific measures [14, 40].

We have analyzed the new measure's asymptotic distribution and computationally show its tendency to the Gaussian curve. Next, the formal proof has been given. We have first concentrated on the null hypothesis that the two rankings are independent and then we have developed tests to do inference for other values of r_W.

Finally, in the last subsection, we claim that there is a wide range of applications where the weighted correlation coefficient r_W can be used to measure the concordance between two rankings.

Chapter 3
The Weighted Rank Correlation Coefficient r_{W2}

Abstract A new weighted rank correlation coefficient, r_{W2}, has been introduced in Pinto da Costa, Weighted Correlation, 2011, [74] and applied in a bioinformatics context in Pinto da Costa et al., IEEE/ACM Trans Comput Biol Bioinf 8(1):246–252, 2011, [73]. This coefficient is the second of its series, following the coefficient r_W introduced in Pinto da Costa et al., Nonlinear Estimation and Classification, MSRI, 2001 [61], Pinto da Costa and Soares, Australian New Zealand J Stat 47(4):515–529, 2005, [63], Soares et al., JOCLAD 2001: VII Jornadas de Classificação e Análise de Dados, Porto, 2001, [93], which was motivated by a machine learning problem concerning the recommendation of learning algorithms. These coefficients were inspired by Spearman's rank correlation coefficient, r_S. Nevertheless, unlike Spearman's, which treats all ranks equally, these coefficients weigh the distance between two ranks using a linear function of those ranks in the case of r_W and a quadratic function in the case of r_{W2}. In both cases, these functions give more importance to top ranks than lower ones, although r_{W2} has some advantages over r_W as we will see. In some of the applications of weighted correlation, ties can happen naturally; nevertheless, the existing coefficients tend to ignore this situation. We give here the expression of r_{W2} in the case of ties. We present also some simulations in order to compare the three coefficients r_{W2}, r_W, and r_S.

3.1 Introduction

In Chap. 2, we described the weighted rank correlation coefficient that we have introduced in 2001 [61, 93]. This coefficient is,

$$r_W = 1 - \frac{6\sum_{i=1}^{n}(R_i - Q_i)^2(2n + 2 - R_i - Q_i)}{n^4 + n^3 - n^2 - n},$$ (3.1)

where R_i is the rank corresponding to the ith observation of the first variable, X, and Q_i is the rank corresponding to the ith observation of the second variable, Y. A deeper study of this coefficient was presented in [63] and explained in Chap. 2, where the sampling distribution was analyzed; in particular, the sampling distribution of r_W converges to the Gaussian as the sample size increases. In addition, the formal

© The Author(s) 2015
J. Pinto da Costa, *Rankings and Preferences*,
SpringerBriefs in Statistics, DOI 10.1007/978-3-662-48344-2_3

proof of this convergence for both dependent and independent data, using a different strategy from [28], was also presented. Our strategy consists of extending the work of [83] to the case of bivariate score functions [67].

In 2003, [28] presented a symmetrized version of Blest's coefficient, $v(X, Y)$, whose expression $(v(X, Y) + v(Y, X))/2$ is equal to

$$\frac{2n+1}{n-1} - \frac{6}{n^2-n}\left(\sum_{i=1}^{n}\left(1 - \frac{R_i}{n+1}\right)^2 Q_i + \sum_{i=1}^{n}\left(1 - \frac{Q_i}{n+1}\right)^2 R_i\right). \quad (3.2)$$

The coefficient r_W was constructed as is usual in such cases by finding an affine function of the distance between the two vectors of ranks that is in the interval $[-1, 1]$. In our case, we wanted to favor the first ranks and so we choose the weighted distance $\sum_{i=1}^{n}(R_i - Q_i)^2(2n + 2 - R_i - Q_i)$.

The construction of Blest's coefficient (and its symmetrized version) is quite different and is based on a graphical approach. Although these constructions and expressions (3.1) and (3.2) are quite different, we have realized that if we simplify them we get the same result; thus, as Genest and Plante pointed out, r_W can also be considered as the symmetrized version of Blest's coefficient [29].

We think that the construction and expression of r_W is not only more clear than the symmetrized version of Blest's coefficient, but also more suitable for generalization.

In Eq. (3.1) (see also [63]), the calculation of the distance between two ranks R_i and Q_i is given by $WD_i^2 = (R_i - Q_i)^2 (2n + 2 - R_i - Q_i)$, where the second term of the product is a linear weighting function which represents the importance of R_i and Q_i. Now, we propose the dissimilarity measure

$$W_2D_i^2 = (R_i - Q_i)^2 (2n + 2 - R_i - Q_i)^2,$$

which reflects more than WD_i^2 the higher importance of agreement on top ranks. In fact, in some circumstances a linear weight function, whose weights belong to $\{2, 3, \ldots, 2n\}$, might not discriminate sufficiently between the different weights. It is common to define rank correlation coefficients, such as Spearman's, as an affine function of the distance between the two vectors of ranks [60]. In our case, this corresponds to define a coefficient of the form

$$a + b\sum_{i=1}^{n}(R_i - Q_i)^2 (2n + 2 - R_i - Q_i)^2. \quad (3.3)$$

In order to find the values of a and b, we will force this function to take the maximum value when the two vectors of ranks are the same ($R_i = Q_i$) and the minimum value when they are the exact opposite of each other ($Q_i = n + 1 - R_i$). As correlation coefficients usually take values in $[-1, 1]$, the first condition ($R_i = Q_i$) implies $a = 1$. Before imposing the second condition in order to find the value of b, let us introduce a different strategy (see also [64]). We will start by defining the transformed (weighted) ranks,

$$R'_i = R_i \, (2n + 2 - R_i) \quad \text{and} \quad Q'_i = Q_i \, (2n + 2 - Q_i).$$ (3.4)

Theorem 2 *Pearson's correlation coefficient of the transformed rankings R' and Q' is equal to* $1 - \frac{90 \sum_{i=1}^{n}(R_i - Q_i)^2 \{2(n+1) - (R_i + Q_i)\}^2}{n(n-1)(n+1)(2n+1)(8n+11)}.$

Proof Given that the sample average of the two vectors of transformed ranks is

$$\gamma(n) = \frac{1}{n} \sum_{1}^{n} R'_i = \frac{1}{n} \sum_{1}^{n} Q'_i = \frac{(n+1)(4n+5)}{6},$$ (3.5)

the value of Pearson's correlation of R' and Q' is

$$\frac{\sum_{i=1}^{n} \left[(R_i \, (2n+2-R_i) - \gamma(n)) \cdot (Q_i \, (2n+2-Q_i) - \gamma(n)) \right]}{\sqrt{\sum_{i=1}^{n} (R_i \, (2n+2-R_i) - \gamma(n))^2} \sqrt{\sum_{i=1}^{n} (Q_i \, (2n+2-Q_i) - \gamma(n))^2}}.$$

When no ties occur in the marginal ranks, this expression simplifies to that of

$$r_{W2} = 1 - \frac{90 \sum_{i=1}^{n} (R_i - Q_i)^2 \{2(n+1) - (R_i + Q_i)\}^2}{n(n-1)(n+1)(2n+1)(8n+11)}.$$ (3.6)

We obtained thus a measure of the form (3.3) that we were looking for, with $a = 1$ and $b = \frac{-90}{n(n-1)(n+1)(2n+1)(8n+11)}$. The weighted correlation coefficient r_{W2} is then Pearson's correlation coefficient of the transformed ranks R' and Q'. This is an important advantage of r_{W2}, compared to other weighted correlation coefficients, because by doing a simple transformation to the data, we can use r_{W2} in any statistical methodology/software that uses Pearson's correlation coefficient.

We can observe that r_{W2} can be written in yet another form, using the expression for the distance measure $W2D_i^2$ above:

$$r_{W2} = 1 - \frac{D_{W2n}}{E(D_{W2n})},$$

where

$$D_{W2n} = \frac{1}{n} \sum_{i=1}^{n} (R_i - Q_i)^2 \, (2n + 2 - R_i - Q_i)^2$$ (3.7)

and

$$E(D_{W2n}) = \frac{n(n-1)(n+1)(2n+1)(8n+11)}{90n}$$

is the expected value of D_{W2n} under independence.

As was noted in [64], for the natural order $R_i = Q_i$, $D_{W2n} = 0$ and so r_{W2} takes the maximum value, that is 1. It can also be seen in Appendix A.2 that the minimum value of this coefficient, that is the maximum value of the distance $\sum_{i=1}^{n} (R_i - Q_i)^2 (2n + 2 - R_i - Q_i)^2$, is attained when the two vectors of ranks are inverted, that is, $Q_i = n + 1 - R_i$, $\forall i = 1, 2, \ldots, n$. The minimum value of r_{W2} obtained is thus,

$$1 - \frac{90 \sum_{i=1}^{n} (R_i - Q_i)^2 (2n + 2 - R_i - Q_i)^2}{n(n-1)(n+1)(2n+1)(8n+11)} = 1 - \frac{90 \sum_{i=1}^{n} (2R_i - (n+1))^2 (n+1)^2}{n(n-1)(n+1)(2n+1)(8n+11)}.$$

This expression simplifies to

$$a = -\frac{14n^2 + 30n + 19}{16n^2 + 30n + 11} > -1$$

This means that the weighted coefficient r_{W2} takes values in the interval $[a, 1]$ (which, as n increases, approaches $[-\frac{14}{16}, 1]$) and not $[-1, 1]$ as is common with correlation coefficients. This is not an original situation. For instance, multivariate versions of Spearman's rho and Kendall's tau coefficients are presented in [55] where the maximum value is not $+1$. We can certainly with an affine transformation force the coefficient r_{W2} to take values in $[-1, 1]$. For that purpose, we recommend the version

$$\tilde{r}_{W2} = \frac{2 r_{W2}}{1 - a} - \frac{1 + a}{1 - a}. \tag{3.8}$$

Let us think now about the meaning of r_{W2} minimum value $a > -1$. It tells us that the perfect positive dependence case ($R_i = Q_i$) is a "stronger" situation than the perfect negative dependence case ($R_i = n + 1 - Q_i$). We think this makes sense because of the weights; for instance, if we swap the same two positions of ranking Q in both cases (perfect positive dependence and perfect negative dependence) the differences in the coefficient will not be the same. Put in another way, we have seen that r_{W2} is Pearson's correlation coefficient of the transformed (weighted) ranks $R_i' = R_i(2n + 2 - R_i)$ and $Q_i' = Q_i(2n + 2 - Q_i)$. Now, when $R_i = Q_i$, the pair (R_i', Q_i') is on a straight line with positive slope; however, when $R_i = n + 1 - Q_i$, the pair (R_i', Q_i') is not on a straight line with a negative slope, although it is not far from it.

As r_W, the coefficient r_{W2} gives more importance to top ranks than lower ones. The idea of giving more importance to the first ranks came from some motivating applications, like algorithm recommendation, where the first positions are more important. We can generalize that application and in order to be able to apply the coefficients r_W and r_{W2}, we rank the data according to our needs. For instance, if we prefer to give more importance to the largest values, we rank the largest value of all as 1, the second largest as 2, and so on. On another situation, as in microarray data, if the largest absolute values are the most important, we give rank 1 to the maximum of gene expressions (in absolute value), rank 2 to the second largest absolute gene expression value, and so on.

In the next section we show that, unlike all other weighted measures, r_{W2} allows to build an explicit formula corrected for ties in the marginal ranks, which is a frequent scenario in some applications. This correction for ties introduced in [64] was derived by using a methodology analogous to the one employed in [45] in order to find the formula for Spearman's coefficient corrected for ties.

3.2 The Formula of the Coefficient r_{W2} in the Case of Ties

We will now show in this section how to compute the value of r_{W2} in the case of ties. This can be a common situation in some of the applications described above and, to the best of our knowledge, no other weighted correlation coefficient works properly in the case of ties in the ranks. This correction for ties, introduced in [64], was derived by using a methodology analogous to the one employed by Kendall [45] in order to find the formula for Spearman's coefficient corrected for ties.

First of all, let us calculate the variances of the transformed ranks

$$V_{R'} = \frac{1}{n} \sum_{i=1}^{n} \left[R_i \left(2n + 2 - R_i \right) - \gamma(n) \right]^2, \tag{3.9}$$

$$V_{Q'} = \frac{1}{n} \sum_{i=1}^{n} \left[Q_i \left(2n + 2 - Q_i \right) - \gamma(n) \right]^2. \tag{3.10}$$

For a set of untied ranks, we have $V_{R'} = V_{Q'} = \frac{n(n-1)(n+1)(2n+1)(8n+11)}{180n}$. In Appendix A.7 we prove that it is possible to write r_{W2} as

$$r_{W2} = \frac{1}{2} \frac{V_{R'} + V_{Q'} - D_{W2n}}{\sqrt{V_{R'}} \sqrt{V_{Q'}}}. \tag{3.11}$$

We will now use this alternative expression in order to obtain a formula of r_{W2} corrected for ties in the marginal ranks. First, we shall adopt the midrank method; that is, we replace the ranks where ties exist by the average of these ranks. For instance, if we observe ties in the second, third, and fourth ranks, we replace those ranks by $\frac{2+3+4}{3} = 3$. We note that when ties occur in the marginal ranks, an application of formula (3.6) for r_{W2} presented above is not the best choice to evaluate the agreement between the two rankings. Suppose, for instance, the following rankings:

$$\begin{array}{llllll} \text{A} & 1.5 & 1.5 & 3 & 4 & 5 & 6 \\ \text{B} & 6 & 5 & 4 & 3 & 1.5 & 1.5 \end{array}$$

In this situation, if we use formula (3.6), we get $r_{W2} = -0.78$. In this formula we use the denominator, $\sqrt{V_{R'}} \cdot \sqrt{V_{Q'}} = \frac{n(n-1)(n+1)(2n+1)(8n+11)}{180n}$, as for the untied form of r_{W2}. However, if there are sets of ties in the two rankings, we note that the quantities $V_{R'}$ and $V_{Q'}$ are reduced and, thus, we need to do a correction. As another, more extreme, example, consider the following rankings: $R = (2, 2, 2)$ and $Q = (1, 2, 3)$. It is clear in this situation that there is no sense in computing a correlation value, it is not defined, since one of the ranks is constant. Nevertheless, if we apply formula (3.6) here, we get $r_{W2} = 0.48$. This obviously does not make sense and so we must correct this formula when ties are present. We will now see the difference ties make in the calculations of the variances $V_{R'}$ and $V_{Q'}$.

Proposition 1 *Suppose, generally, that t ranks $R_k + 1, \ldots, R_k + t$ in the first ranking are tied. Then, the variance of the transformed rankings R' becomes*

$$\grave{V}_{R'} = \frac{n(n-1)(n+1)(2n+1)(8n+11)}{180n} - \frac{1}{n}\left[\frac{t - t^2 - t^3 + t^4}{3} + \frac{2n(t - t^3)}{3}\right]$$

$$\times R_k - \frac{1}{n}\left[\frac{t^3 - t}{3}\right]R_k^2 - \frac{1}{n}\left\{\frac{t^2}{6} - \frac{nt}{3} - \frac{11t}{180} - \frac{t^3}{36} - \frac{t^4}{6} + \frac{4t^5}{45} + \frac{nt^2}{3}\right.$$

$$\left. - \frac{n^2t}{3} + \frac{nt^3}{3} - \frac{nt^4}{3} + \frac{n^2t^3}{3}\right\}.$$

Proof Taking ties into account in the first ranking, the summation part in (3.9) corresponding to the t tied ranks for the calculation of $V_{R'}$ will be composed of t terms all containing the average transformed rank given by

$$\frac{1}{t}\sum_{j=1}^{t}\left[(R_k + j)(2n + 2 - (R_k + j))\right]$$

$$= \left(R_k + \frac{t+1}{2}\right)(2n + 2)$$

$$- \left(R_k^2 + (t+1)R_k + \frac{(t+1)(2t+1)}{6}\right).$$

If we ignore the ties, we use in this summation the t different terms $(R_k + j)(2n + 2 - (R_k + j)), j = 1, 2, \ldots, t$. Let us now see the difference between the two cases in summation (3.9):

$$\sum_{j=1}^{t}\left[(R_k + j)(2n + 2 - (R_k + j))\right]^2$$

$$- t\left\{\left(R_k + \frac{t+1}{2}\right)(2n + 2) - \left(R_k^2 + (t+1)R_k + \frac{(t+1)(2t+1)}{6}\right)\right\}^2$$

$$= \left[\frac{t - t^2 - t^3 + t^4}{3} + \frac{2n(t - t^3)}{3}\right]R_k$$

$$+ \left[\frac{t^3 - t}{3} \right] R_k^2 + \frac{t^2}{6} - \frac{nt}{3} - \frac{11t}{180} - \frac{t^3}{36} - \frac{t^4}{6} + \frac{4t^5}{45}$$

$$+ \frac{nt^2}{3} - \frac{n^2t}{3} + \frac{nt^3}{3} - \frac{nt^4}{3} + \frac{n^2t^3}{3}.$$

It is therefore this quantity that we have to subtract in order to correct the variance of ranking R'.

Suppose now that we have various sets of ties in the first ranking ($R_k + 1, \ldots, R_k + t$ for various values of k and t) and also in the second ranking ($Q_l + 1, \ldots, Q_l + u$ for various values of l and u). Then, by applying Proposition 1, the variances of the transformed rankings R' and Q' after correction become

$$\grave{V}_{R'} = \frac{n(n-1)(n+1)(2n+1)(8n+11)}{180n} - \frac{\grave{T}_{W2}}{n},$$

and

$$\grave{V}_{Q'} = \frac{n(n-1)(n+1)(2n+1)(8n+11)}{180n} - \frac{\grave{U}_{W2}}{n},$$

where

$$\grave{T}_{W2} = \sum_t \left[\left(\frac{t - t^2 - t^3 + t^4}{3} + \frac{2n(t - t^3)}{3} \right) R_k + \left(\frac{t^3 - t}{3} \right) R_k^2 \right.$$
$$\left. + \left(\frac{t^2}{6} - \frac{tn}{3} - \frac{11t}{180} - \frac{t^3}{36} - \frac{t^4}{6} + \frac{4t^5}{45} + \frac{nt^2}{3} - \frac{n^2t}{3} + \frac{nt^3}{3} - \frac{nt^4}{3} + \frac{n^2t^3}{3} \right) \right],$$

and

$$\grave{U}_{W2} = \sum_u \left[\left(\frac{u - u^2 - u^3 + u^4}{3} + \frac{2n(u - u^3)}{3} \right) Q_k + \left(\frac{u^3 - u}{3} \right) Q_k^2 \right.$$
$$\left. + \left(\frac{u^2}{6} - \frac{un}{3} - \frac{11u}{180} - \frac{u^3}{36} - \frac{u^4}{6} + \frac{4u^5}{45} + \frac{nu^2}{3} - \frac{n^2u}{3} + \frac{nu^3}{3} - \frac{nu^4}{3} + \frac{n^2u^3}{3} \right) \right].$$

Here, $\sum_t$ and $\sum_u$ stands for summation over various sets of ties in the first and second rankings, respectively.

Based on this, and similarly to what was done by Kendall [45] to correct the variance of Spearman's coefficient in the presence of ties, we will now replace $V_{R'}$ and $V_{Q'}$ by $\grave{V}_{R'}$ and $\grave{V}_{Q'}$, respectively, and we obtain the expression of the coefficient in the presence of ties:

$$r_{W2} = \frac{1}{2} \frac{\grave{V}_{R'} + \grave{V}_{Q'} - D_{W2n}}{\sqrt{\grave{V}_{R'}} \sqrt{\grave{V}_{Q'}}}. \tag{3.12}$$

We note that when there are no ties, $\dot{U}_{W2} = \dot{T}_{W2} = 0$ and this last expression reduces to (3.11). If we use this corrected expression in the first example above, we obtain $\dot{U}_{W2} = \dot{T}_{W2} = \frac{121}{2}$ and $r_{W2} = -0.91$. This value is quite different from the uncorrected one, -0.78, and it expresses higher disagreement between the two rankings. If we use this corrected expression in the second example above, the value will be undefined, as it should, since $\dot{V}_{R'} = 0$.

As we have seen the modifications that the presence of ties have in Eq. (3.6) are quite complex. One can always do the easiest, which is to use Pearson's correlation coefficient of the weighted ranks R' and Q' (see Eq. (3.4)), after adopting the midrank method. This gives us an approximate value. When there are no ties, we can do the same or use instead formula (3.6).

Finally, if we prefer to use the version $\tilde{r}_{W2}$ (3.8) that takes values in $[-1, 1]$, we just have to first correct the value of r_{W2} and then make the transformation above (3.8).

We present next a simulation study in order to compare the three coefficients r_{W2}, r_W and r_S.

3.3   Comparison Between the Three Coefficients r_{W2}, r_W and r_S

In this section, we will compare the new weighted correlation coefficient, r_{W2}, with the previous coefficient r_W and also with Spearman's coefficient, as in [64]. Despite the similarities between the three measures r_{W2}, r_W and r_S, they may yield quite different values when applied to the same pair of series. We illustrate these differences using a few examples. We measure the correlation between rankings $\mathbf{R}$ and $\mathbf{Q}$. The former is defined as $\mathbf{R} = (1, 2, \ldots, n - 1, n)$, where n is the number of elements in the ranking. Ranking $\mathbf{Q}$ is obtained from $\mathbf{R}$ by swapping the elements $(1, \ldots, p)$ and $(q - p + 1, \ldots, q)$, after inverting the order in each of them:

$$\mathbf{R} = \quad (\boxed{1, \ldots, p}, p + 1, \ldots, q - p, \boxed{q - p + 1, \ldots, q}, q + 1, \ldots, n)$$

$$\mathbf{Q} = (\boxed{q, \ldots, q - p + 1}, p + 1, \ldots, q - p, \boxed{p, \ldots, 1}, \quad q + 1, \ldots, n).$$

We plot in Fig. 3.1 the value of $r_{W2}(\mathbf{R}, \mathbf{Q}) - r_W(\mathbf{R}, \mathbf{Q})$ for a few values of n, p and q. The figure shows that the two measures yield values that are quite different, especially taking into account that the values of p used in this experiment are relatively small when compared to n. This means that, the differences in the weighted correlations measures, using the two coefficients, obtained for larger values of p would be greater.

Furthermore, Fig. 3.2 shows that the new coefficient, r_{W2}, provides even more weight to the top ranks than r_W because the differences to the unweighted correlation, r_S, are greater (see also [63] and the last chapter).

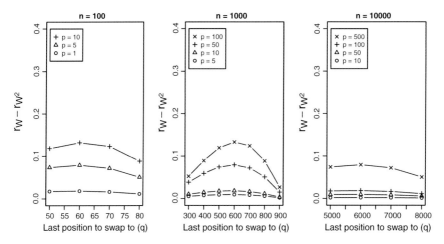

Fig. 3.1 Difference between the previously proposed weighted measure of correlation (r_W) and the new one (r_{W2}) on a few illustrative examples

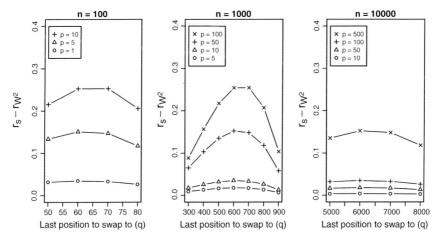

Fig. 3.2 Difference between Spearman's coefficient (r_S) and the new weighted measure of correlation (r_{W2}) on a few illustrative examples

We conclude that the new coefficient, r_{W2}, is even more appropriate than its predecessor, r_W, for applications where top ranks are more important than lower ones. Like r_W, r_{W2} gives more importance to top ranks. This is done while still taking the whole ranking into account rather than simply assuming that some ranks matter and others do not.

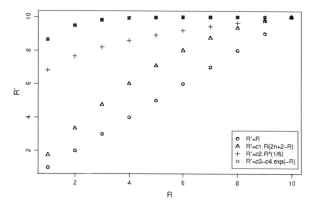

Fig. 3.3 Scatterplot for four different rank transformations

3.4 A New Way of Developing Weighted Correlation Coefficients

Compared to r_W, the weighted correlation coefficient r_{W2} has the additional advantage that it is equal to the Pearson correlation coefficient of the transformed ranks $R'_i = R_i(2n + 2 - R_i)$ and $Q'_i = Q_i(2n + 2 - Q_i)$. This is a very important advantage because any method/software that uses Pearson's correlation coefficient, can from now on use r_{W2} instead, after the appropriate data transformation has been realized. This means also that we can use it when there are tied values, by contrast with r_W; we just have to use average ranks when there are ties and then apply Pearson's correlation to the transformed ranks R'_i and Q'_i.

The coefficient r_{W2} made us look at the problem of weighted correlation from a different perspective (see also [74]). In fact, by applying a transformation to the ranks so that the first ones are favored and then computing Pearson's correlation coefficient of the transformed ranks, we can define many new measures of weighted correlation. In Fig. 3.3, we can see four different cases. The first, when $R' = R$, corresponds to Spearman's coefficient and so it does not correspond to a weighted measure; when $R' = R(2n + 2 - R)$ we have r_{W2}. We can now use other functions such as $R' = R^{1/6}$ or $R' = -e^{-R}$. In order to be able to represent the four cases in the same diagram, we had to multiply some of the transformations by a constant and in the last case also add another constant; however, these operations do not change the value of Pearson's correlation. Thus, the importance given to the first ranks is larger when $R' = -e^{-R}$ and smaller when $R' = R$.

By approaching the problem from this perspective, all that is needed is that the transformation is monotonic and the last ranks are more flattened by the transformation compared with the first ranks. Naturally, other types of transformations can be used if we want to favor other ranks.

Chapter 4
A Weighted Principal Component Analysis, WPCA1; Application to Gene Expression Data

Abstract In this chapter, we describe in the first part new developments in Principal Component Analysis (PCA) Jolliffe, Principal Component Analysis, 2002, [42] and in the second part a new method to select variables. The focus is on problems where the values taken by each variable do not all have the same importance and where the data may be contaminated with noise and contain outliers, as is the case with microarray data. This kind of data, which contains the expression levels of a large number of genes (variables), measured simultaneously, for a relatively much smaller number of tissue samples, presents many statistical challenges. The usual PCA is not appropriate to deal with this kind of problem. In this context, we propose the use of a weighted correlation coefficient as an alternative to Pearson's. This leads to a so-called weighted PCA (WPCA1). In order to illustrate the features of this WPCA1 and compare it with the usual PCA, we consider the problem of analyzing gene expression datasets. In the second part of this chapter, we propose a new PCA-based algorithm to iteratively select the most important genes in a microarray dataset. We show that this algorithm produces better results when WPCA1 is used instead of the usual PCA. Furthermore, using the well-known supervised classification method of Support Vector Machines, we show that this algorithm can also compete with the Significance Analysis of Microarrays (SAM) supervised algorithm, Tibshirani et al., Diagnosis of multiple cancer types by shrunken centroids of gene expression. PNAS, 10, 1999, [97] and Tusher et al., Proc Nat Acad Sci, 98:5116–5121, 2001, [98].

4.1 Introduction

In this chapter, we describe in the first part new developments in Principal Component Analysis (PCA) [42] and in the second part a new method to select variables. The focus is on problems where the values taken by each variable do not all have the same importance and where the data may be contaminated with noise and contain outliers, as is the case with microarray data. This kind of data, which contains the expression levels of a large number of genes (variables), measured simultaneously, for a relatively much smaller number of tissue samples (for instance, tumor tissues), presents many statistical challenges. The usual PCA is not appropriate to deal with

© The Author(s) 2015
J. Pinto da Costa, *Rankings and Preferences*,
SpringerBriefs in Statistics, DOI 10.1007/978-3-662-48344-2_4

this kind of problems. In this context, we propose the use of a weighted correlation coefficient as an alternative to Pearson's. This leads to a so-called weighted PCA (WPCA1). In order to illustrate the features of this WPCA1 and compare it with the usual PCA, we consider the problem of analyzing gene expression datasets. In the second part of this chapter, we propose a new PCA-based algorithm to iteratively select the most important genes in a microarray dataset. We show that this algorithm produces better results when WPCA1 is used instead of the usual PCA. Furthermore, using the well-known supervised classification method of Support Vector Machines, we show that this algorithm can also compete with the Significance Analysis of Microarrays (SAM) supervised algorithm [97, 98].

PCA is a dimensionality reduction method which consists of finding a smaller number of variables, which are a linear combination of the original variables, of decreasing importance. PCA is thus widely used in the analysis of high-dimensional data. There are, however, some applications where the usual PCA is not recommended because it gives the same importance to all of the observations and is sensitive to the presence of outliers and noise in the data. For instance, the larger absolute expression values in microarrays should be given higher importance as they relate to genes that are more "responsible" for the problem in analysis. Basically, the amount of expression of a gene indicates the approximate number of copies of mRNA of that gene which are produced inside the cell, and so it provides information about the gene function and contribution to the development of the related problem [13, 34, 90]. In addition, as pointed out in [85], a gene which has a lower expression level in one condition will typically be measured with relatively less precision in that condition, and so these expression values can be very noisy.

In this chapter (see also [72, 73]), we propose,

- First, a new PCA to solve the aforementioned problems affecting the usual PCA. In order to cope with outliers and noise, we will use rankings instead of the original data. For instance, in microarray data, we will start by ranking the expression values (observations) in each gene (variable). Then, in order to give higher weight to the larger absolute expression values inside each gene, we will use the new weighted rank correlation coefficient, introduced in [73], instead of the usual Pearson's. This gives rise to a so-called weighted PCA (WPCA1).
- Second, a new PCA-based algorithm to iteratively select the most important genes for discriminatory purposes in a microarray dataset.

We will illustrate the application of WPCA1 to microarray data because this kind of data possesses all the characteristics that we need to illustrate the method presented in this chapter. We have searched for works that give higher importance to the larger expression values in PCA, but there are only a few. For instance, Jansen et al. [41] use an established method of weighted PCA introduced in [48] to weigh the elements of metabolomics data in accordance with a priori information. The problem of robustness to outliers and noise is also of major importance (see, for instance, [38, 102]); however, the usual PCA and the weighted PCA of [48] do not cope with it. Finally, the PCA-based algorithms for selecting the most important genes in microarrays, like the one in [24], take into account the importance of each principal component in an isolated fashion, and highly correlated genes can be chosen as being important, which can add redundancy to the process of gene selection.

In this chapter, we begin by describing in Sect. 4.2 a novel weighted PCA based on a new rank correlation coefficient. Moreover, we illustrate its features and apply it to microarray data. Next, in Sect. 4.5, we describe a PCA-based algorithm for selecting the most important variables for discriminatory purposes in a dataset. We compare the classification results using Support Vector Machines [16] in microarray datasets for four different methods of choosing genes: our algorithm with WPCA1, our algorithm with the usual PCA, the popular SAM supervised algorithm [97, 98], and an unsupervised algorithm called Pattern discovery via eigengenes [97, 98]. Furthermore, we explain the biological meaning of the relevant genes chosen. Finally, we end the chapter in Sect. 4.6 with the main conclusions.

Before moving on, we note that although the application focused on here concerns microarray experiments, a broader range of applications can be considered. As an example, we can look at problems containing preferences stated by humans or recommendations provided by decision support systems; naturally, the first preferences or recommendations are more important and accurate than the last ones. Another potential application of the WPCA1 methodology is when we have various stock trading support systems and we want to summarize the information given by them. In this case what investors want is a grading of the stocks in question, which can be represented by a ranking. If we have various rankings corresponding to different support systems, we might want to summarize the information using PCA; however, the stocks ranked higher can be more important than the last ones. Another problem that is usually handled as a ranking task is information retrieval [4]. Again, rank importance should be taken into account, although that rarely happens [40]. Similar remarks apply to recommender systems [14].

4.2 A New Weighted Version of PCA

Our aim in this section is to develop a new PCA methodology in order to reduce the dimension of the input space, which is a major problem in many applications nowadays, as is the case of microarray data just described. We seek thus for a few linear combinations of the variables that account for most of the variations present in the data. This is done using PCA, introduced by Karl Pearson in 1901 and Hotelling in 1933 [34, 42]. Let us denote by $\mathbf{X} = (X_1, X_2, \ldots, X_p)^T$ the vector containing all measurements for the p variables (genes in microarray data). Thus, our data consists of n vectors $\mathbf{X}_1, \mathbf{X}_2, \ldots, \mathbf{X}_n$ in a space of p dimensions, where n is the number of samples. Mathematically, the PCA problem consists of finding a subspace of dimension K of the original space which maximizes the dispersion of the points projected onto that subspace. The solution to this optimisation problem (see [34, 51]) is given by the eigenvectors corresponding to the K largest eigenvalues of the covariance matrix of the sample, $\hat{\Sigma} = \frac{1}{n} \sum_{i=1}^{n} (\mathbf{X}_i - \hat{\mu})(\mathbf{X}_i - \hat{\mu})^T$, where $\hat{\mu}$ is the mean vector of the sample. For various reasons, it is common to start by standardizing the data. This consists of subtracting from each observation the average of the variable in question and divide by the corresponding standard deviation times $\sqrt{n}$. With this initial standardization, the principal components obtained are linear combinations of the standardized variables, and the coefficients of these linear combinations are given by the elements of the eigenvectors of the usual correlation matrix based on Pearson's correlation coefficient, r.

In the usual PCA, the eigenvectors of the covariance matrix or the Pearson correlation matrix (standardized data) contain the coefficients of the linear combinations of the original variables corresponding to the new variables (features, components). As is well known, the Pearson correlation coefficient is very sensitive to the presence of outliers and noise. To overcome this, we will use the ranks of the observations. We must therefore start by ranking the observations in each variable from 1 (highest rank) to n (lowest rank). For the sake of simplicity, let us use the ranks directly rather than the values in the series, that is, R_i and Q_i to represent the ranks of two variables (genes in our application) corresponding to observation (sample) i. Now, if we calculate Pearson's correlation coefficient of the ranked data, we obtain the Spearman's rank correlation coefficient, r_S, which is given by the expression

$$r_S = \frac{\sum_{i=1}^{n} \left(R_i - \overline{R}\right)\left(Q_i - \overline{Q}\right)}{\sqrt{\sum_{i=1}^{n} \left(R_i - \overline{R}\right)^2 \sum_{i=1}^{n} \left(Q_i - \overline{Q}\right)^2}},$$

where $\overline{R}$ and $\overline{Q}$ are the average ranks. However, for computational purposes, a more convenient expression which assumes there are no ties is

$$r_S = 1 - \frac{6 \sum_{i=1}^{n} (R_i - Q_i)^2}{n^3 - n}.$$

Here, we introduce a weighted version of PCA (WPCA1), where more importance is given to observations whose values are more important. We think this makes sense for instance with microarray data, given that, as explained in Sect. 4.1, the higher the absolute expression value the more probable that the gene in question is related to the particular problem. To that end, this weighted PCA uses a new correlation coefficient that gives higher weights to observations that are considered to be more important. In addition, this correlation coefficient is not sensitive to the presence of outliers and noise in the data.

4.3 Preliminary Version of Weighted Principal Component Analysis Using r_W

A preliminary version of weighted PCA has been introduced in [65, 69], where we used a different weighted rank correlation coefficient introduced in [63] (see also Chap. 2),

$$r_W = 1 - \frac{6\sum_{i=1}^{n}(R_i - Q_i)^2 (2n + 2 - R_i - Q_i)}{n^4 + n^3 - n^2 - n} \qquad (4.1)$$

The application that we consider here concerns the problem of selecting informative genes from the thousands of genes whose expression is usually measured in microarray experiments. We approach the problem by finding the Principal Components of the most expressed genes. PCA is a well-known technique of data analysis that is very popular in Bioinformatics. For instance, a quick search for "Principal Component Analysis" shows thousands of occurrences only in the web page of the Bioinformatics journal, which attests to the popularity of this technique. Two variants are used: the usual PCA using the Pearson correlation matrix and a "weighted" version which was introduced in [65, 66] and later improved [73]. This "weighted" PCA consists of using an adaptation of a new rank correlation coefficient that gives more importance to higher ranks and which was introduced by Pinto Costa & Soares in [61, 63, 93].

Our aim now is to use the two correlations (Pearson's r and "weighted" r_W) as inputs for the PCA and compare the results obtained. First of all, because we have many more variables (genes) than observations (samples) in the considered datasets, we will start by filtering the genes that we think are most important. This is done by considering only the most expressed genes. Second, we apply the "weighted" and unweighted PCA to the chosen genes and find the new variables, corresponding to the principal components, which are a linear combination of the chosen genes. These principal components have been called "eigengenes" [95]. Then, as suggested in [24], suppose that for instance the first principal component is $\sum a_i x_i$, where the a_i are the coefficients in that component and x_i is the expression level for gene i. Restricting attention to those genes for which $|a_i| > c$, for some chosen cutoff value c, allows us to focus on a small set of genes that might be used in a future microarray experiment, for instance.

We considered five different datasets containing gene expression from samples (instances) having or not one of possibly various forms of cancer (classes), obtained from the url http://www.lsi.us.es/~aguilar/datasets.html and another url http://www-stat.stanford.edu/~tibs/ElemStatLearn/data.html. The datasets are identified as follows: Colon cancer (2 classes: 1—Tumor, 2—Normal); Embryonal tumors (of the central nervous system) (2 classes: 1—Tumor, 2—Normal); Global cancer map (14 classes: 1—Breast, 2—Prostate, 3—Lung, 4—Colorectal, 5—Lymphoma, 6—Bladder, 7—Melanoma, 8—Uterus Adeno, 9—Leukemia, 10—Renal, 11—Pancreas, 12—Ovary, 13—Mesothelioma, 14—CNS); Leukemia (2 classes: 1—ALL, 2—AML); NCI (14 classes: 1—CNS, 2—Renal, 3—Breast, 4—NSCLC, 5—Unknown, 6—Ovarian, 7—Melanoma, 8—Prostate, 9—Leukemia, 10—K562B-repro, 11—K562A-repro, 12—Colon, 13—MCF7A-repro, 14—MCF7D-repro). For each of the datasets, the 15 most expressed genes were used in the usual (Pearson's r) and in the "weighted" (r_W) PCA. Figure 4.1 shows the cumulative explained variance for a number of principal components, i.e., eigengenes, ranging from 1 to 15, and two major conclusions are drawn: although the

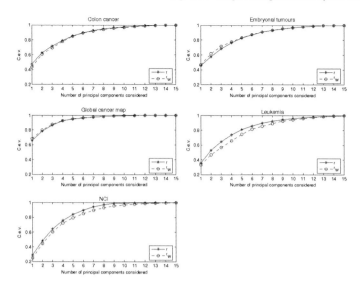

Fig. 4.1 Cumulative explained variance (C.e.v.) for each of the approaches to PCA—usual (Pearson's r) and "weighted" (r_W)—in the five datasets

eigengenes are different, the cumulative explained variance is almost the same in both approaches to PCA; apart from the Global cancer map dataset, the minimum number of eigengenes needed to explain at least 80 % of the total variance is about 5. The usual (Pearson's r) and a "weighted" (r_W) PCA were used to select both the so-called eigengenes, a compressed representation of gene expression through principal components, and the most important genes in some of the most important eigengenes. Most of the times, the two forms of PCA selected different genes or the same genes but in a different order of importance; nevertheless, we observed that the associated eigengenes explain almost the same total variance of gene expression. Given that the results obtained with this weighted version of PCA were not very different from the usual PCA, we explored another weighted version of PCA, which we describe next.

4.4 Weighted Principal Component Analysys, WPCA1, Using r_{W2}

The coefficient r_W used in our preliminary version of PCA has nevertheless some drawbacks,

- It cannot be used when there are tied values; its expression was based on Spearman's expression for untied values;
- In some applications, a linear weighting function might not be enough;

- We did not succeed in writing r_W as an inner product, which is a useful property for PCA as we will see.

In this section we will use the weighted correlation coefficient r_{W2}, described in Chap. 3, and whose expression,

$$
r_{W2} = \frac{\sum_{i=1}^{n} \left(R_i' - \overline{R'} \right) \left(Q_i' - \overline{Q'} \right)}{\sqrt{\sum_{i=1}^{n} \left(R_i' - \overline{R'} \right)^2} \sqrt{\sum_{i=1}^{n} \left(Q_i' - \overline{Q'} \right)^2}},
$$

has been given in [68]. We propose to use it in PCA.

It is clear from Chap. 3 that the computation of the correlation coefficient r_{W2} is equivalent to doing a data transformation on each variable as

$$
R_i' = R_i \left(2n + 2 - R_i \right), \tag{4.2}
$$

and then compute the Pearson correlation coefficient. R_i represents the rank of each observation value; usually the smallest value has rank 1, the second smallest rank 2, and so on. However, depending on the problem, we can rank the observations differently. For instance, in microarray data, because we want to give higher weight to the larger absolute expression values and r_{W2} gives higher weights to the first ranks, we will therefore give rank 1 to the largest absolute value, rank 2 to the second largest, etc.

We can see therefore that if we start by ranking and then transforming our data according to (4.2) for each variable in the dataset, then the application of the usual normed PCA uses the weighted correlation coefficient r_{W2}. We note therefore that the weighted PCA can be done using any common software for PCA analysis. If in our dataset the number of variables is smaller than the number of observations that is all that we have to do. Otherwise, it is common to use Singular Value Decomposition (SVD) or the NIPALS algorithm [100]. However, we describe in Appendix— Sect. A.8 a simpler yet efficient way for computing the principal components whenever there are more variables than observations in the data.

In bioinformatics, a common application of PCA is on the analysis of the high-dimensional microarray data. As pointed out by Bicciato et al. [6], molecular diagnostics based on microarray data present major challenges due to the overwhelming number of variables and the complex, multiclass nature of tumor samples. Thus, it is of paramount importance to have the development of both suitable automatic marker selection methods, like those based on PCA, that allow the identification of genes that are most likely to confer high classification accuracy of multiple tumor types, and suitable multiclass classification schemes. The works in [32, 85] are also examples of the use of PCA for gene expression data analysis. Naturally, other types of data in bioinformatics can be analyzed by this powerful technique. For instance, Jansen et al. [41] use PCA to get a simplified view of metabolomics data. Scholz et al. [89] apply PCA, but also independent component analysis, to detect relevant

Table 4.1 Datasets used in the practical experiments

Dataset	Samples	Genes
Embryonal tumors	60	7129
Global cancer map	144	16063
Leukemia	38	7129
NCI60	64	6830

information from spectra of total compositions of metabolites. Many more examples could be given to show the importance of PCA in these and other applications in bioinformatics.

In the following, we will apply our method to four microarray datasets, namely those described in Table 4.1.[1]

Our aim now is to compare results when we apply the usual PCA and our WPCA1. We recall that in order to apply WPCA1, we only need to consider as input data to a PCA software the original data transformed according to (4.2).

4.4.1 Robustness to Outliers and Noise

As discussed in the introduction, the presence of noise in microarray data is common and that motivated us to use ranks instead of the original data to cope with this problem. We will now design an experiment to show that, first of all, outliers are very common in this kind of data and then we will use both the usual PCA and our weighted version to see how much outliers affect them. Let us denote by $\xi_{0.25}$ and $\xi_{0.75}$ the first and third quartiles of the expression values for a given gene. We will use a common criterion which considers that all observations outside the interval $[\xi_{0.25} - 1.5(\xi_{0.75} - \xi_{0.25}), \xi_{0.75} + 1.5(\xi_{0.75} - \xi_{0.25})]$ are outliers and those outside $[\xi_{0.25} - 3(\xi_{0.75} - \xi_{0.25}), \xi_{0.75} + 3(\xi_{0.75} - \xi_{0.25})]$ severe outliers. In the four datasets under consideration the number of genes containing outliers of the two types are described in Table 4.2.

We see therefore that in the first two datasets more than 90 % of the genes contain outliers and around 65 % in the third and fourth datasets. Also, inside the genes containing outliers, we found that around 6 % of the observations, on average, are outliers. Thus, as suspected, there are many outliers which we will show that affect the usual principal component analysis, given that it is based on Pearson's correlation coefficient which is very sensitive to outliers. We will now pick a small number of genes in order to illustrate the effect outliers have in the two correlations (Pearson's r and ours r_{W2}) and then compute the two principal component analyses before and after the removal of outliers to see how robust they are. We will use genes g19, g600,

---

[1] http://www.lsi.us.es/~aguilar/datasets.html, http://www-stat.stanford.edu/~tibs/ElemStatLearn/data.html.

Table 4.2 Number of genes containing outliers and severe outliers in the four datasets

Dataset	Number of genes	Number of genes with outliers	Number of genes with severe outliers
Embryonal tumors	7129	6672	3553
Global cancer map	16063	15893	13073
Leukemia	7129	4713	1504
NCI60	6830	4421	788

Table 4.3 Values of r and r_{W2} for the genes g19, g600, and g830 in the Embryonal tumors dataset, before and after the removal of all outliers

Before removal of all outliers			
Correlation	(g19, g600)	(g19, g830)	(g600, g830)
r	0.7113	−0.5593	−0.6883
r_{W2}	0.6198	0.5463	0.6563
After removal of all outliers			
Correlation	(g19, g600)	(g19, g830)	(g600, g830)
r	0.6597	0.4696	0.4984
r_{W2}	0.5395	0.4458	0.5953

g830 of the first dataset, Embryonal Tumors, in our example which have 3, 5, and 6 outliers, respectively. Table 4.3 contain the values of r and r_{W2} for these three genes before and after the removal of all outliers.

As is clear from these tables, the effect of outliers in Pearson's correlation is dramatic; for instance, for the genes g19 and g830, before the removal of outliers the correlation was −0.5593 and after the removal of outliers was 0.4696! The values of r_{W2} also change, because we have removed some observations; but, as is clear, the differences before and after the removal are much smaller. To finalize this section, we will now find the expression of the first two principal components, which account

Table 4.4 Expression of the first two principal components for the genes g19, g600, and g830 in the Embryonal tumors dataset, before and after the removal of all outliers

r		
PC1	Before	$0.0053 \times g19 + 0.9411 \times g600 - 0.3381 \times g830$
	After	$0.0042 \times g19 + 0.8740 \times g600 + 0.4859 \times g830$
PC2	Before	$0.0139 \times g19 + 0.1763 \times g600 + 0.9842 \times g830$
	After	$0.0023 \times g19 + 0.6691 \times g600 - 0.7432 \times g830$
r_{W2}		
PC1	Before	$0.5615 \times g19 + 0.5960 \times g600 + 0.5740 \times g830$
	After	$0.5468 \times g19 + 0.5933 \times g600 + 0.5908 \times g830$
PC2	Before	$-0.7708 \times g19 + 0.1247 \times g600 + 0.6248 \times g830$
	After	$-0.8320 \times g19 + 0.3661 \times g600 + 0.4169 \times g830$

for around 90 % of the total variation in all four cases. We shall do that first for the situation before the removal of outliers and then for the situation after the removal of outliers to analyze the differences (Table 4.4).

As we suspected, large differences occur in the expression of the principal components when we use the usual PCA (correlation r); the importance (coefficient) given to the three genes changes sometimes drastically when we remove the outliers. As for our weighted WPCA1 (correlation r_{W2}) the changes are comparatively small, as we expected.

Thus, the inclusion of the outliers, which are very important observations in this problem, has a dramatic effect as it can change completely the results: if we do not include the outliers and include only the other observations, the results can be opposite, so to say. This is not a desirable property of the usual correlation or PCA; we do not want to ignore the outliers because in this application they represent certainly important information about the problem; nevertheless, we would like that the difference in the final results was not so large. Our correlation r_{W2} is thus appropriate to this problem because it gives higher importance (weight) to the outlier observations which is very appropriate here; nevertheless, it is much more robust because including the outliers does not change dramatically neither the values of the correlation nor the principal components.

Up to now we described a novel weighted PCA and showed its relevance in analyzing gene expression data. In the remainder of the chapter, we will focus on choosing relevant genes for the datasets under analysis here.

4.5 A New Method for Selecting Relevant Genes in Microarray Data

In the previous sections, we learned how to find the principal components, both for the usual and the weighted PCAs. Here, we propose a new PCA-based algorithm for selecting the most important genes for discriminatory purposes in a microarray dataset, which is an important problem [20, 23, 97]. The idea is to filter the genes most associated with the conditions (diseases) in each dataset that we will analyze. We compare the obtained results, in the four microarray datasets above, using Support Vector Machines (SVMs) which is a classification algorithm whose aim is to predict the type of disease using the genes selected. Four different methods of choosing genes will be used: our algorithm with WPCA1, our algorithm with the usual PCA, the popular SAM supervised algorithm [97, 98], and an unsupervised algorithm called Pattern discovery via eigengenes (here PDeig for short) [97, 98].

In any PCA, each of the principal components is a linear combination of all of the variables present in the dataset; usually thousands of them. This makes it very difficult to interpret each principal component. Suppose that, for instance, the first principal component was $\sum a_i X_i$, where a_i are the coefficients in that component and X_i represents the values of variable i. It has been suggested [24] that restricting attention to those variables for which $|a_i| > c$, for some chosen cutoff value c, allowed us to focus on a small set of variables that might contain the most important information. However, this brings four problems. First, as is usually known, the principal components have not all the same importance and so, should not be treated in the same way. Second, the variables which appear in all of the principal components (PCs) are the same and so we have to analyze all of the PCs at the same time and not separately. Third, in case of supervised classification problems, we want our selection procedure to take into account the discriminant power of each gene. Fourth, many of the variables in the dataset are highly correlated and in order to choose a good and small list of genes we should prioritize uncorrelated genes; as Tibshirani et al. [97] pointed out, after a minimal list is found, one can always search for more genes that are highly correlated with the genes in that list. In our experiments using SVMs, we have found better discriminatory results by prioritizing uncorrelated genes. This is also found by Dudoit et al. [23, p. 85] in some of their experiments.

In order to solve the problems just mentioned, we introduce here a strategy for choosing the L most important original variables after a PCA (usual or weighted) has been performed on the dataset. The number L must be chosen by the user. The first thing we have to do is to decide how many principal components to use. There are many ways to choose the number of principal components, K, and here we will choose as many as needed to have at least 90 % of the information present in the dataset. Thus, we can represent each of the K principal components by

$$\mathrm{PC}_k = \sum_{i=1}^{p} a_{ki} X_i, \quad k = 1, \dots, K, \qquad (4.3)$$

where X_i represents variable i and a_{ki} the coefficient given by the kth principal component to that variable. Let us denote by λ_k the importance of the kth component, which corresponds to an eigenvalue of a certain matrix, as seen above. We will now define the global importance of each variable X_i, $i = 1, 2, \dots, p$, by the expression

$$\mathrm{GI}(X_i) = DP(X_i) \times \sum_{k=1}^{K} |a_{ki}| \lambda_k, \qquad (4.4)$$

where $DP(X_i) = \dfrac{s_{\bar{X}_i}^2}{\sum_k s_{X_i^k}^2}$, which is the ratio between the variance of the class centers and the sum of the variances within each class, which allows us to take into account the discriminant power of the variable X_i (see the third problem above). Now, in order to find the L most important variables, we apply the next algorithm,

1. Choose the variable X_i which maximizes the global importance given by Eq. (4.4). This is the most important variable of all.
2. Now, for $l = 1, 2, \dots, L - 1$ do

a. For each variable X_i not yet chosen, find the Pearson correlation coefficient between X_i and the l variables which have already been chosen: $r(X_i, X_j)$, $j = 1, \ldots, l$. Let $r_{\max,i}$ be the maximum in absolute value of these l correlations.

b. Actualise the global importance of variable X_i by

$$\text{GI}^\star(X_i) \;=\; \text{GI}(X_i) \times (1 - r_{\max,i}). \qquad (4.5)$$

c. Choose the variable X_i which maximizes the actualised global importance given by Eq. (4.5).

4.5.1 Support Vector Machines Classification: Results for Genes Chosen with SAM, PDeig, and with Our Method for WPCA and PCA

In this section, we will compare the genes selected by the weighted PCA with those chosen by the usual PCA in terms of discriminatory power. Furthermore, we will show that our method of selecting genes is very competitive with the popular supervised method called SAM and better than an unsupervised method called PDeig. The data concerning the genes selected by the four methods are used as inputs to the SVMs software included in R [77], namely in the e1071 library. We used the default parameters in R for tuning the SVMs with the sigmoid and radial basis kernels, that is, for the sigmoid kernel $\mathscr{K}(u, v) = \tanh(\gamma u^T v + c)$ we set $\gamma = 1/(\text{data dimension})$ and $c = 0$, and for the radial basis kernel $\mathscr{K}(u, v) = \exp(-\gamma ||u - v||^2)$ we took $\gamma = 1/(\text{data dimension})$.

Given that all four methods have parameters which influence the number of genes to choose, for comparison purposes we will use the same number of genes in the four cases. In the Embryonal tumors dataset, SAM chose 16 genes by default and so we used the same number of genes in the WPCA1 and PCA methods. In the other three datasets, SAM chooses hundreds of genes by default; however, in our experiments, we found that the classification results with such a large number of genes are not significantly better than considering only 20 genes. This type of behavior was also observed in [23, p. 85] and pointed out in [2], where the authors conclude that the number of genes can be reduced greatly without increasing the prediction error.

Table 4.5 presents the mean classification error rate obtained with tenfold cross-validation. It can be seen that in the first, second, and fourth datasets WCPA1 is better than PCA and PDeig and very competitive with SAM. The third dataset is very simple in what concerns discriminating between the classes and so three methods exhibit very good results, namely WPCA1, PCA, and SAM, whereas the other method, PDeig, has a poorer performance.

Table 4.5 Support vector machines error results

Dataset	SVM kernel	WPCA	PCA	SAM	PDeig
Embryonal tumors	Sigmoid	0.17	0.20	0.18	0.37
	Radial basis	0.20	0.22	0.17	0.35
Global cancer map	Sigmoid	0.47	0.51	0.62	0.68
	Radial basis	0.42	0.45	0.61	0.68
Leukemia	Sigmoid	0.00	0.00	0.03	0.20
	Radial basis	0.00	0.00	0.03	0.18
NCI60	Sigmoid	0.18	0.23	0.54	0.66
	Radial basis	0.27	0.25	0.49	0.56

4.5.2 Analysis of the Chosen Genes

In this section, we will study the biological relevance of some of the most important genes used in Sect. 4.5.1. We will restrict our attention to the genes chosen by WPCA1, PCA, and SAM, given that the results obtained by PDeig are comparatively poor.

In the Embryonal tumors dataset, the leukotriene C4 synthase *LTC4S* (gene U50136rna1) and the neurotrophic tyrosine kinase, receptor, type 3 (TrkC) *NTRK3* (gene S76475) are identified both by SAM and our WPCA1-based algorithm. Mutations in *NTRK3* have been associated with medulloblastomas, secretory breast carcinomas and other cancers (see [75]). Furthermore, our method includes the hi,gh mobility group AT-hook 1 *HMGA1* (gene L17131rna1), the Sodium channel 2 mRNA (gene hBNaC2) ,and the alternatively spliced *ACCN2* (gene U78180), which were not identified by SAM as being relevant; these genes are also referred in [75].

In the Global cancer map dataset, the ARHGDIB Rho GDP dissociation inhibitor (GDI) beta *ARHGDIB* (gene L20688) is identified by both SAM and our WPCA1-based algorithm. Moreover, our method includes the KLK3 kallikrein-related peptidase 3 *KLK3* (gene X07730) and the vascular endothelial growth factor C *VEGF-C* (gene U43142), which were not identified by both SAM and the usual PCA-based algorithm. The first gene is in the Kallikreins subgroup of serine proteases, which have diverse physiological functions. Growing evidence suggests that many kallikreins are implicated in carcinogenesis and some have potential as novel cancer and other disease biomarkers (see http://www.ncbi.nlm.nih.gov/sites/entrez). In turn, the second gene is essential in lymph node metastasis, presumably because enhanced metastatic potential including lymphangiogenesis induced by VEGF-C is vital in lymph node metastasis of gastric cancer [49].

In the Leukemia dataset, SAM and our WPCA1-based algorithm identified six genes in common. Some of the remainder genes identified by our method include the cell division cycle 25 homolog A *CDC25A* (gene M81933), *SMARCA4* (gene D26156s), the interleukin 18 *IL*-18 (gene D49950), the myb myeloblastosis viral oncogene homolog (avian) *MYB* (gene U22376cds2s), the Non-SMC condensin I complex, subunit D2 *NCAPD2* (gene D63880), and the CUG triplet repeat, RNA binding protein 1*CUGBP1* (gene U63289). *CDC25A* is overexpressed in a variety of human malignancies [101]; inactivating mutations of the *SMARCA4* gene, on chromosome *arm19p*, are present in several human cancer cell lines [54]; interleukin 18 *IL*-18 establishes a possible functional relationship between IL-18 and MMPs in myeloid leukemia; myb myeloblastosis viral oncogene homolog (avian) *MYB* is overexpressed in most human acute myeloid and lymphoid leukemias, and several studies using antisense oligonucleotides and dominant negative forms of *MYB* have shown that this gene activity is essential for continued proliferation of AML and CML cells; *CUGBP1* is involved in the development of breast cancer and leukemia (see [59]). The three selection methods found homeobox A9 *HOXA9* (gene U82759) as a relevant gene, which is in fact important for leukemia identification [25].

In the NCI60 dataset, the genes *CD53* antigen and *DKK3* dickkopf homolog 3 (Xenopus laevis) 2 were identified by all three methods. *CD53* antigen interactions might contribute to cell survival in poorly vascularized regions of the tumor mass [103]. In turn, *DKK3* can play a role in head and neck squamous cell carcinoma (HNSCC) carcinogenesis with unknown mechanism [43]. The genes laminin, alpha 3 *LAMA3*, and paxillin *PXN* were identified by both WPCA and PCA, but not by SAM. Downregulation of Laminin-5 (LN5)-encoding genes (*LAMA3*, *LAMB3* and *LAMC2*) has been reported in various human cancers [86]. Furthermore, the results in [86] demonstrate epigenetic inactivation of LN5-encoding genes in breast cancers and association of *LAMA3* promoter methylation with increased tumor stage and tumor size. On the other hand, in lung cancer tissues [39], for paxillin *PXN* an important role has been established. Finally, our WPCA1-based algorithm further identified the gene transducin-like enhancer of split 1 (E(sp1) homolog, Drosophila) *TLE1*. This gene was also consistently found by several independent groups to be an excellent discriminator between synovial sarcoma and other sarcomas, including histologically similar tumors such as malignant peripheral nerve sheath tumor [96].

4.6 Conclusions

In this chapter, we used a new correlation coefficient that weighs observations according to their importance to the problem in hand and which is robust to the presence of outliers and noise in the data. Then, we proposed the use of this weighted correlation coefficient on principal component analysis, and concluded that its application to PCA is equivalent to doing a certain data transformation. This gave rise to a novel weighted PCA, WPCA1, which is more robust than the usual PCA in microarray datasets.

We described also a new algorithm to select the most important variables in the original dataset to which a PCA, usual or weighted, is applied. This PCA-based algorithm takes into account the global importance of each component, the discriminatory power of each variable and does not add redundancy by disabling the selection of new variables that are highly correlated with previously chosen ones. We verified in some microarray datasets that our PCA-based algorithm produces better results when our WPCA1 is used instead of the usual PCA. Furthermore, we showed that it can compete with the popular Significance Analysis of Microarrays (SAM) algorithm. The classifiers using the data corresponding to the genes chosen by these three methods were built using Support Vector Machines. The classification results were supported by the biological meaning of the relevant genes chosen.

Chapter 5
A Weighted Principal Component Analysis (WPCA2) for Time Series Data

Abstract Time series are ubiquitous in all fields of application. In some situations, the number of observations in each series is too large and so it is of paramount importance to be able to compress the series reducing thus its dimension. One very popular method for both dimensionality reduction and feature extraction is Principal Component Analysis (PCA). The classical PCA gives the same importance to all of the variables. However, in a time series context, it is frequent that some observation times are more important than others. In order to take this into account, a weighted PCA specific for time series data, which was introduced in Pinto da Costa, J., Silva, I., Silva, M.E., IASC 07 (book of abstracts): Statistics for data mining, learning and knowledge extraction, page 32 (2007), is described in this chapter. The method is applied to well-known datasets and the results are compared with those obtained by classical PCA.

5.1 Introduction

Time series are ubiquitous in all fields of application. In some situations, the number of observations in each series is too large and so it is of paramount importance to be able to compress the series reducing thus its dimension. One very popular method for both dimensionality reduction and feature extraction is Principal Component Analysis (PCA). The classical PCA gives the same importance to all of the variables. However, in a time series context, it is frequent that some observation times are more important than others and should therefore be given larger weight in the analysis. These weights will be input into the distance between two time series by means of a weighted correlation. As noted in the introduction, weighted correlation is concerned with the use of weights assigned to the subjects in the calculation of a correlation coefficient between two variables X and Y. The weights can either be naturally available beforehand or chosen by the user to serve a specific purpose.

In order to take into account the weights given to each observation time for time series PCA, a weighted PCA specific for time series data, which was introduced in [70], is described in this chapter. The method is applied to well-known datasets consisting of multidimensional time series and the results are compared with those

© The Author(s) 2015
J. Pinto da Costa, *Rankings and Preferences*,
SpringerBriefs in Statistics, DOI 10.1007/978-3-662-48344-2_5

obtained by classical PCA. Multidimensional time series and space-time series are now common. In many situations, the number of observations in each series is too large and thus it is very important to extract the most important information and discarding noise and redundant correlations by means of PCA. This is also useful for graphical representation and for future statistical analysis of the time series data. PCA delivers a new set of variables, called principal components, that are uncorrelated and ordered so that the first few retain most of the variation presented in the dataset [42]. Formal inference procedures on principal components rely on the independence of the observations as well as on multivariate normality. However, correlated datasets such as multidimensional time series and space–time series are becoming the norm rather than the exception. Moreover in some statistical analysis, namely in cluster analysis, the objective is to look for dependence within the dataset thus obtaining useful insights of its structure [50]. Therefore, when the purpose of the analysis is descriptive, not inferential, correlation among the observations is not a hindering issue for PCA [42].

Usually, PCA gives the same importance to all of the variables. However, in a time series context, it is obvious that some of the observations should play a leading role. For instance, consider the values of two stocks in a stock exchange market over the previous year. An assessment of their similarity may be important, for instance, in order to decide whether to buy. In this case, the most recent behavior is clearly more relevant. In other applications, like feature extraction for discriminant analysis, it may be that in some parts of the series the classes are very well separated and in other parts not so much. Here, it would be advantageous to give higher weight to the observation times where the classes are well separated and smaller weight elsewhere. In other situations, it can be useful to consider that certain parts of the time series should have no influence at all (zero weight). Thus, depending on the objective of the analysis, we need to define an appropriate weight function in order to proceed.

The aim of this chapter is to propose a weighted PCA, WPCA2, specific for time series data that gives more weight to some of the observations. To our knowledge, there is no other method of weighted PCA for time series data. There has been a very limited number of works on weighted PCA for other types of data. For instance in [73], the authors focus on problems where the values taken by each variable do not all have the same importance and where the data may be contaminated with noise and contain outliers, as is the case with microarray data. They introduce a weighted PCA by using the weighted correlation coefficients introduced in [63, 68, 73]. In [41], the authors use an established method of weighted PCA introduced in [48] to weight the elements of metabolomics data.

5.2 Motivation and Definition

The principal components were introduced by Karl Pearson in 1901 and Hotelling in 1933 (see [34]). PCA aims at reducing the dimension of the feature space by means of a linear transformation. Mathematically, the problem consists of finding a subspace of the original space which maximizes the dispersion of the points projected onto that subspace. If a small number of principal components explains a large portion of the variance of the original variables, then PCA can be used as a dimension reduction technique.

Let $\{\mathbf{y}_1, \mathbf{y}_2, \ldots, \mathbf{y}_n\}$, $\mathbf{y}_i \in \mathbb{R}^p$, $i = 1, \ldots, n$, be a set of n time series, each one with p observations, corresponding to n observations on a p-dimensional space, that can be represented by the following $(n \times p)$ matrix:

$$\mathbf{Y} = \begin{bmatrix} \mathbf{y}_1 \\ \mathbf{y}_2 \\ \vdots \\ \mathbf{y}_n \end{bmatrix} = \begin{bmatrix} y_{\bullet 1}, y_{\bullet 2}, \ldots, y_{\bullet p} \end{bmatrix} = \begin{bmatrix} y_{11} & y_{12} & \cdots & y_{1p} \\ y_{21} & y_{22} & \cdots & y_{2p} \\ \vdots & \vdots & \ddots & \vdots \\ y_{n1} & y_{n2} & \cdots & y_{np} \end{bmatrix}. \tag{5.1}$$

When we consider the space determined by the point values of the time series, we will have a cloud of n points (time series) in $\mathbb{R}^p$ and we aim at reducing the number of variables, corresponding to the p observations of each of the time series. As is usually the case, the p variables $y_{\bullet j}$ are highly correlated and so a feature extraction method appropriate for time series data is most useful. PCA is a powerful and very popular method of feature extraction which is very useful when the variables are very correlated, as is the case here. However, the usual PCA treats all of the p variables $y_{\bullet j}$ in the same way; that is, it gives the same importance (weight) to all of them. In many applications of time series, it is obvious that the most recent observations should have a larger influence like for instance data from the stock exchange markets. Given the values of two stocks over the last year and if we want, for instance, to see how similar they are in order to decide whether to buy, their most recent behavior can be much more important than the initial values. In order to give higher weight to the most recent observations in the feature extraction procedure, we will describe here a novel method of Weighted PCA that is especially designed for time series data [70]. However, its application to other types of data is straightforward.

Let now $\mathbf{X}$ be the matrix of the centered data, i.e., $\mathbf{X} = [x_{ij}]$, $x_{ij} = y_{ij} - \overline{y}_{\bullet j}$, $i = 1, \ldots, n$; $j = 1, \ldots, p$ where $\overline{y}_{\bullet j} = \frac{1}{n} \sum_{i=1}^{n} y_{ij}$ is the mean value for time j. The ith row of matrix $\mathbf{X} = \begin{bmatrix} \mathbf{x}_1 & \mathbf{x}_2 & \ldots & \mathbf{x}_n \end{bmatrix}^p = \begin{bmatrix} X_1 & X_2 & \ldots & X_p \end{bmatrix}$ is the transformed ith time series.

The principal components are therefore new variables, which are a linear combination of the initial p variables corresponding to the p values of the time series. The coefficients of these linear combinations are given by the elements of the eigenvectors of the usual covariance matrix. Thus, to obtain the usual principal components, the matrix $\mathbf{S} = \mathbf{X}^T \mathbf{X}$ must be diagonalized. $\mathbf{S}$ is a multiple of the covariance matrix and may not have full rank. In this case, it is usual to use singular value decomposition (SVD) or the NIPALS algorithm [100], which runs faster than SVD. Here a simpler and well-known strategy is used, which consists in diagonalizing $\mathbf{X}\mathbf{X}^T$ instead, thus obtaining the eigenvalues of $\mathbf{X}\mathbf{X}^T$, which are the same as the eigenvalues of $\mathbf{X}^T \mathbf{X}$. If x is a unit eigenvector of $\mathbf{X}\mathbf{X}^T$ and λ the corresponding eigenvalue, then $\frac{1}{\sqrt{\lambda}} \mathbf{X}^T x$

is a unit eigenvector of the matrix $\mathbf{X}^T\mathbf{X}$ (with eigenvalue λ). Note that if $p > n$ at least the last $p - n + 1$ eigenvalues are zero; here, only the nonzero eigenvalues are considered.

Let $(\lambda_1, \boldsymbol{v}_1), (\lambda_2, \boldsymbol{v}_2), \ldots, (\lambda_p, \boldsymbol{v}_p)$ be the (eigenvalue, eigenvector) pairs of $\mathbf{S}$, where $\lambda_1 \geq \lambda_2 \geq \cdots \geq \lambda_p$ and $||\boldsymbol{v}_i|| = 1$. Then the jth principal component is defined by $Z_j = \mathbf{X}\boldsymbol{v}_j = v_{j1}X_1 + v_{j2}X_2 + \cdots + v_{jp}X_p$, $j = 1, \ldots, p$, with $\mathrm{Var}(Z_j) = \lambda_j$, $j = 1, \ldots, p$. The total variance of the data is given by $\lambda_1 + \cdots + \lambda_p$. The proportion of total variance due to the jth principal component is $\lambda_j / \left(\lambda_1 + \cdots + \lambda_p\right)$, $j = 1, \ldots, p$. There are many methods to help choose the number M of principal components that represent the data with enough accuracy. In this work, M will be the number of principal components that explain at least 90 % of the variability present in the data.

As is well known, in PCA we have always to start by centering the variables:

$$x_{ij} \leftarrow (x_{ij} - \overline{x}_{\bullet j}); \tag{5.2}$$

then to define the distance between objects (time series) we have to arm $\mathbb{R}^P$ with an Euclidean metric associated with a positively defined matrix. The most common matrices are the identity and also $D_{\frac{1}{s^2}}$, which is a diagonal matrix whose components are the inverses of the p variances of the columns $s_{\bullet 1}^2, s_{\bullet 2}^2, \ldots, s_{\bullet p}^2$; $s_{\bullet j}^2 = \frac{1}{n}\sum_{i=1}^n (x_{ij} - \overline{x}_{\bullet j})^2$. This matrix is used especially when the variables are measured in very different scales, in order to avoid that variables which are not relevant but have larger variance dominate the analysis. The use of this diagonal matrix is equivalent to doing an initial operation after centering the observations which consists of reducing them by dividing by the corresponding standard deviation:

$$x_{ij} \leftarrow \frac{y_{ij} - \overline{y}_{\bullet j}}{s_{\bullet j}}, \tag{5.3}$$

and then using the usual Euclidean distance. The final result will be that if we apply this operation to our data, the PCA will need to find the eigenvectors and eigenvalues of the Pearson correlation matrix. This is known as normed PCA. Inspired by this standardization, which gives higher weight to the variables presenting smaller variance, we introduced in [70] other data transformations that suit our needs.

In Eq. (5.3) each centered variable is multiplied by a weight, $\frac{1}{s_{\bullet j}}$. The variables whose influence we want to reduce are multiplied by smaller weights; the others by a larger weight. This is similar to what we want to do here, that is, to give higher weight to some variables and smaller to others. However, these weights, $\frac{1}{s_{\bullet j}}$, are not needed in our case because in our time series data all variables (observation times) are of the same type. Nevertheless, we were inspired by this transformation (5.3) to introduce a weighted version of PCA, WPCA2, specific for time series data (see [70]). For instance, instead of multiplying by $1/s_{\bullet j}$, the centered variables may be multiplied by other weights $\sqrt{w_j}$:

$$x_{ij} \leftarrow \sqrt{w_j}\,(y_{ij} - \overline{y}_{\bullet j}) \tag{5.4}$$

where $w_j \geq 0$ and, for comparison purposes, $\sum_{j=1}^{p} w_j = 1$. For instance, in the normed PCA just discussed, $w_j = 1/s_{\bullet j}^2$, where $s_{\bullet j}^2$ is the variance of the jth column of the matrix $\mathbf{X}$.

After transforming the data according to (5.4), the usual PCA is applied, which means that a weighted matrix of covariances, that is, the usual covariances after transforming the data according to (5.4), will be diagonalized. Thus, the WPCA2 procedure discussed here requires an adequate selection of weights, depending on the objective of the analysis. For instance, if we want to give higher importance to the most recent observations, we will use weights like $w_j = j$, $w_j = j^2$ and $w_j = \alpha^j$, for a suitable choice of α. If we want to favor other observations, we just have to choose an appropriate weight function.

When we use transformation (5.3), then the covariance matrix that we have to diagonalize is a multiple of the usual Pearson correlation matrix. By using transformation (5.4), we will get a weighted matrix of covariances. In fact, we could have used the Euclidean distance associated with the matrix $D_w = \mathrm{diag}(w_j)$, which is a diagonal matrix whose elements are the weights. As for the previous case, the use of this Euclidean distance is equivalent to applying transformation (5.4) and then using the usual Euclidean distance.

After this initial data transformation, any common software for PCA can be used.

5.3 Weight Functions: Examples

The choice of an appropriate weight function to be used in practice depends on the purpose of the analysis. If the recent observations are considered the most important, then linear ($f_j = a + bj$), quadratic ($f_j = a + bj^2$), or exponential ($f_j = a^j$) weight functions may be entertained. It is important to note that for these functions, the actual weights, w_j, depend not only on the type of weight function, but also on the length of the time series. For instance, with a linear weight function the weight given to the first observation is $w_1 = \frac{a+b}{\sum_{j=1}^{p}(a+bj)} = \frac{a+b}{ap+bp(p+1)/2}$, which depends on the length, p. This problem is overcome by introducing another parameter, γ, which is equal to the relative importance of the last observation (the most important in this example) to the first observation (the least important):

$$\gamma = \frac{f_p}{f_1}. \tag{5.5}$$

Thus, if the last observation is to have an influence in the analysis, say, ten times larger than the first, then $\gamma = 10$. The values used in this chapter are $\gamma = 2, 10, 100$.

From the above, it follows that the actual weights (normalized weights) are given by

$$w_j = \frac{f_j}{\sum_{h=1}^{p} f_h},$$ (5.6)

where the values of f_j satisfying (5.5) can be:

$$f_j = \frac{p - \gamma^2}{p - 1} + \frac{(\gamma^2 - 1)}{p - 1} j, \quad \text{for the linear case}$$ (5.7)

$$f_j = \frac{p^2 - \gamma^2}{p^2 - 1} + \frac{(\gamma^2 - 1)}{p^2 - 1} j^2, \quad \text{for the quadratic case, and}$$ (5.8)

$$f_j = a^j, \quad \text{where} \quad a = \exp\left(2 \frac{\ln(\gamma)}{p - 1}\right), \quad \text{for the exponential case}$$ (5.9)

These are the weight functions that we have used when the last observations of the times series are to be given higher importance than the first observations. We will now see another situation. Consider, for instance, the problem of feature extraction for discriminant analysis [26, 36, 37]. Suppose that each of the n time series $\{y_1, y_2, \ldots, y_n\}$ in Eq. (5.1) belongs to one of K predefined classes. In order to assess the discriminatory power of $y_{\bullet j}$, the observational variable at time j, $j = 1, 2, \ldots, p$, the following criterion is defined:

$$d_j = \frac{\sum_{c=1}^{K} n_c (\overline{y}_{j_c} - \overline{y}_{\bullet j})^2}{\sum_{c=1}^{K} s_{j_c}^2},$$ (5.10)

where n_c is the number of time series belonging to the cth class, $\overline{y}_{\bullet j} = \frac{1}{n} \sum_{i=1}^{n} y_{ij}$ is the total average of all time series at instant j, $\overline{y}_{j_c} = \frac{1}{n_c} \sum_{i=1}^{n_c} y_{j_{ci}}$ and $s_{j_c}^2 = \frac{1}{n_c} \sum_{i=1}^{n_c} (y_{j_{ci}} - \overline{y}_{j_c})^2$ are, respectively, the usual sample mean and sample variance of the values of the time series belonging to the cth class at instant j. The larger the value of d_j the higher the discriminatory power of instant j. Then, the weights to be used in this situation are as follows:

$$w_j = \frac{d_j}{\sum_{h=1}^{p} d_h}.$$ (5.11)

5.4 Applications

In this section, we will start by applying our WPCA2 in order to analyze some time series datasets, namely two datasets from the UCR Time Series Data Mining Archive [46], "reality check" and "18 pairs", that has been used in [99] and another dataset that has been used in [17]; see also [70]. "Reality check" consists of 14 time series of normalized data, each with 1,000 data points taking values in the range [0,1], from space shuttle telemetry, exchange rates, and artificial sequences. The "18 pairs" dataset contains 36 time series with 1,000 data points which come in pairs (18 pairs thus). The third dataset consists of 20 time series indices with 309 data points, from January 1977 to September 2002, about the Industrial Production (by Market Group) indices in the United States (source: http://www.economagic.com). This dataset has originated two other datasets: the one used in Caiado et al. [17], which contains a specific transformation ($y_{ij} = \log(x_{ij}) - \log(x_{i(j-1)})$) and another one containing normalized values in the range [0,1] ($y_{ij} = (x_{ij} - \min_{1 \le j \le t}\{x_{ij}\})/(\max_{1 \le j \le t}\{x_{ij}\} - \min_{1 \le j \le t}\{x_{ij}\})$). We have thus five datasets in total.

We will now apply the WPCA2 described above to the five datasets. One of the typical problems in PCA has to do with the number of components to consider. We will choose the M most important principal components that explain at least 95 % of the variance present in the data. For each dataset, we will apply the usual PCA (without weights) and three versions of our weighted PCA, for the linear, quadratic, and exponential weight functions.

In Table 5.1, we present for each dataset the number of components for each case, M, the weight function, the total variance explained, and the variance explained by each of the M most important components.

For the "reality check" dataset, the differences are quite clear. Although the number of components is the same for the three first scenarios, the importance of each component is not; in fact, the importance of the first PC is always increasing from the case of no weight to the exponential weight case. As for the second component, the reverse situation seems to happen, although not so markedly. For the fourth and fifth components, again the situation of the first PC seems to happen. Finally, for the exponential weight case a drastic change happened where only one component seems to be responsible for the variation in the data. This is certainly due to the fact that the last values of the time series are the ones which play a role in the analysis, since the weight given to the majority of the data observations is almost zero. The exponential weight case could be further analyzed in order to find, for each application, the most appropriate value of α.

For the "18 pairs" and the Ind. Prod. (original) datasets, it was not possible to see significant differences among the four scenarios (no weight, linear, quadratic, exponential). This happens because these data are quite simple and so, even for the no weight case, one PC is enough with around 99 % of explained variance. Thus, the weighted cases could not show their power, because it is not possible to get less than one component. This suggests that when the data is already in a one-dimensional space there is not much point in using the weighted PCA.

For the Ind. Prod. (transformed) dataset, a similar situation to the first dataset seems to happen, although with some differences. First of all, the number of components is the same for the no weight and linear weight case, then decreases for the quadratic weight case and decreases again for the exponential weight case. Also, the importance of the first PC increases from the no-weight case to the quadratic weight

Table 5.1 PCA results for each dataset

Dataset	Weight function	M	Total Var. Expl. (%)	Var. Expl. by each PC (%)
Reality check	No weight	5	95.3	33.7; 28.6; 15.6; 9.8; 7.6
	Linear	5	96.0	42.4; 23.2; 16.8; 7.1; 6.5
	Quadratic	5	97.5	52.9; 21.7; 15.1; 5.7; 2.5
	Exponential	1	99.8	99.8
18 Pairs	No weight	1	98.7	98.7
	Linear	1	98.7	98.7
	Quadratic	1	98.7	98.7
	Exponential	1	99.8	99.8
Ind. Prod. (original)	No weight	1	98.2	98.2
	Linear	1	99.5	99.5
	Quadratic	1	99.7	99.7
	Exponential	1	100.0	100.0
Ind. Prod. (transformed)	No weight	8	95.7	50.0; 21.5; 9.0; 6.1; 3.1; 2.5; 1.9; 1.5
	Linear	8	95.8	57.9; 16.4; 8.2; 5.4; 3.1; 1.9; 1.8; 1.2
	Quadratic	7	95.2	62.5; 14.8; 7.1; 4.6; 3.0; 1.7; 1.5
	Exponential	5	96.3	57.1; 21.4; 8.7; 6.4; 2.7
Ind. Prod. (normalized)	No weight	4	96.8	58.3; 29.2; 7.2; 2.2
	Linear	4	96.4	59.2; 25.6; 8.6; 3.0
	Quadratic	4	97.3	47.7; 38.1; 7.0; 4.4
	Exponential	1	96.3	96.3

case, but then decreases for the exponential weight case. The other components have a mixed behavior; sometimes their importance increases, sometimes decreases.

For the Ind. Prod. (normalized) dataset, the situation seems again to differ from the other situations. As is expected, the number of components is either the same, or decreases, when we go from the no-weight case to the exponential weight case. As for the importance of the first PC, a new situation happens. Its importance is similar for the first two cases, then decreases and then increases again substantially.

As is clear from these few examples, large differences can occur with WPCA2. We will now present in Figs. 5.1, 5.2 and 5.3, the scatterplots for the two most important principal components for the cases where it was possible to see a significant difference in Table 5.1.

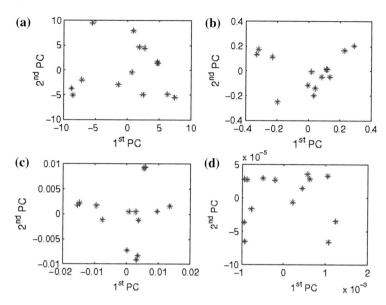

Fig. 5.1 Scatterplots of the two most important PCs of the Reality Check dataset, considering the following weight functions: **a** no weight, **b** linear, **c** quadratic, and **d** exponential

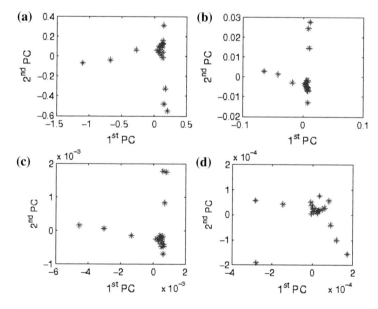

Fig. 5.2 Scatterplots of the two most important PCs of the Industrial Production indices dataset (transformed), considering the following weight functions: **a** no weight, **b** linear, **c** quadratic, and **d** exponential

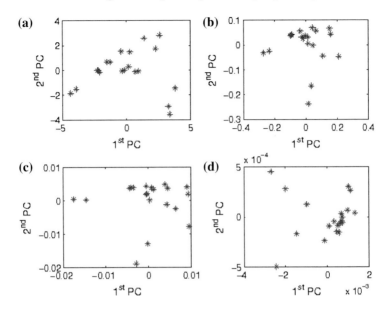

Fig. 5.3 Scatterplots of the two most important PCs of the Industrial Production indices dataset (normalized), considering the following weight functions: **a** no weight, **b** linear, **c** quadratic, and **d** exponential

From the analysis of these figures, it seems clear that not only the importance of the principal plane varies from the no-weight situation to the exponential weight case, but also these planes are different. In fact, the scatterplots change significantly in the four situations, which means that they are in fact different. A deeper study of these results shall illustrate the consequences of WPCA2 in the final proximities observed in the representations: we expect that those time series which are more similar in the last part and not so similar in the first will be closer in the scatterplots than two time series presenting an opposite behavior.

In these five datasets, we have applied a novel method of Weighted PCA, WPCA2, specific for time series data, although its application to other types of data is straight-forward. Our aim so far has been to give higher importance to the most recent observations and we have shown that it was achieved because large differences can occur. We will now deepen this application study, by applying the WPCA2 technique and the classical PCA to five other time series datasets.

Four out of the next five datasets come from the UCR Time Series Classification/Clustering Homepage [47], "Synthetic Control", "FaceAll", "Trace," and "CBF". The other dataset, "d19", belongs to the competition datasets (see site in http://www.cs.ucr.edu/~eamonn/SIGKDD2007TimeSeries.html) of the Workshop and Challenge on Time Series of the 13 th ACM SIGKDD International Conference on Knowledge Discovery and Data Mining Classification (2007).

The "Synthetic Control" (SynthControl) dataset contains 600 time series, each with 60 observations, of six different classes of control charts synthetically generated

Table 5.2 Comparison of the results of PCA and WPCA2 with a discriminant weight function

Dataset	Weight function	M	Var. explained by PC1–PC3 (%)	Total var. explained by PC1–PC3 (%)	Discr. power of PC1
SynthControl	Without discriminant	36	44.61; 5.04; 4.32	53.97	6580.1
		23	57.12; 5.93; 3.09	66.14	5220.9
FaceAll	Without discriminant	32	20.63; 13.95; 7.4	41.98	78.2
		12	60.16; 11.64; 5.13	76.93	715.1
Trace	Without discriminant	4	67.74; 16.76; 4.09	88.59	1829.0
		1	97.1	97.1 (only PC1)	2965.1

by the process described in Ref. [1]. The "FaceAll" dataset is from a face classification problem based on the head profiles (see [79] for details). A number of photos has been taken on 14 individuals making different expressions on the face. Then, each head profile is converted, starting from the throat, into a "pseudo time series" by measuring the local angle of a trace of its perimeter. This dataset contains 2250 time series, with 131 observations each. Note that the "d19" dataset corresponds to the "FaceAll" dataset, but in a reverse time order and so the last observations in "d19" correspond to the profile relating to the mouth and nose, which are considered the most important in this application. This dataset seems therefore appropriate for the weight functions which favor the last observations. The "Trace" dataset is a subset of the Transient Classification Benchmark first introduced in [80]. This is a synthetic dataset designed to simulate instrumentation failures in a nuclear power plant. Similarly to [79], in this work the second feature of class 2 and 6, and the third feature of class 3 and 7 are used. Therefore, there are 200 time series with 275 observations each. The "CBF" dataset has been used for validation of time series classification systems (see [31] for details). There are three classes of objects: Cylinder, Bell, and Funnel (each class is characterized by a specific pattern). This dataset consists of 930 time series with 128 observations. This dataset seems also appropriate for the weight functions which favor the last observations.

Table 5.2 presents, for the "Synthetic Control", "FaceAll," and "Trace" datasets, the results of the classical PCA (without weight function) and WPCA2 with the discriminant weight function. It contains the number of principal components, M, that explain at least 90 % of variability of the data, the variance explained by each of the three most important components (PC1, PC2, and PC3), the total variance explained by these three components and the discriminatory power of the first principal component, given by (5.10).

The results show that, for the three datasets, the number of principal components decreases when discriminant weights are used, allowing higher level of compression of the data. The discriminatory power of PC1 for the "Synthetic Control" dataset decreases when computed by WPCA2 with discriminant weights but presents a huge

Table 5.3 Comparison of the results of PCA and WPCA2 when higher weight is given to the most recent observations

Dataset	Weight function	γ	M	Var. explained by PC1–PC3 (%)	Total var. explained by PC1–PC3 (%)
CBF	Without	–	68	31.7; 10.56; 7.49	49.75
	Linear	2	62	31.24; 12.34; 7.59	51.17
		10	54	31.37; 13.75; 7.49	52.61
		100	54	31.38; 13.82; 7.48	52.68
	Quadratic	2	59	30.68; 12.85; 7.49	51.02
		10	44	31.16; 15.59; 7.07	53.82
		100	42	31.23; 15.76; 7.06	54.05
	Exponential	2	60	30.86; 12.55; 7.56	50.97
		10	36	30.73; 16.34; 6.69	53.76
		100	22	32.78; 16.54; 6.71	56.03
d19	Without	–	32	20.63; 13.95; 7.4	41.98
	Linear	2	25	23.42; 15.86; 8.86	48.14
		10	21	24.74; 16.8; 9.56	51.10
		100	21	24.8; 16.84; 9.59	51.23
	Quadratic	2	24	24.17; 16.51; 9.83	50.51
		10	16	26.35; 18.25; 11.23	55.83
		100	16	26.46; 18.34; 11.3	56.10
	Exponential	2	25	23.78; 16.2; 9.53	49.51
		10	13	26.85; 21.05; 13.03	60.93
		100	8	31.96; 26.02; 13.34	71.32

increase for the other two datasets. For the three datasets, the variance explained by PC1 increases considerably in the weighted situation.

Table 5.3 presents the results for the "CBF" and "d19" datasets applying the classical PCA (without weight function) and WPCA2 with the weight function which gives higher weight to the most recent observations. The γ value, the number of components retained for each case, M, the variance explained by each of the three most important components (PC1, PC2, and PC3) and the total variance explained by these three components are presented. Once again, M decreases as the weight of the most recent observations increases. In addition, for a fixed weight function, the value of M decreases with the increase of the parameter γ which represents the relative importance between the last observation and the first observation. Furthermore, it is evident that using weights makes the three-dimensional space corresponding to the first three principal components more important, since the total variance explained by these three components tends to be larger, in some cases much larger.

5.5 Final Remarks

This chapter describes a method of Weighted PCA, WPCA2, specific for time series data, although its application to other types of data is straightforward. The purpose is to give different weights to the observation times, according to a certain goal. Here the goal is either to favor the observation times which present higher discriminant power or else to favor the most recent observations. Naturally, other types of weights can be used in other situations. The results indicate that the number of principal components needed to explain a fixed proportion of total variance may decrease for WPCA2. Thus, WPCA2 is capable of higher levels of compression of the data. Moreover, the results show that the first principal component obtained from WPCA2 with a discriminant weight function can be more useful to discriminate among the classes. Finally, WPCA2 has the advantage of not requiring any assumptions on the time series under study, such as stationarity, as do other procedures proposed in the literature (see [3]).

Chapter 6
Weighted Clustering of Time Series

Abstract We will describe here a method for the clustering of time series. This method does not give the same importance to all of the observations; instead, it lets the most important observations, for instance the most recent, have a larger weight. A fundamental problem in the clustering of time series is the choice of a relevant metric, and here, we will use a metric, based on Pearson's correlation coefficient, which uses the notion of weighted mean and weighted covariance. We present also some motivating applications.

6.1 Introduction

In this chapter, we consider the problem of clustering time series introduced in [71]. Contrary to other works on this topic, our main concern is to let the most important observations, for instance the most recent, have a larger weight on the analysis. This is done by defining a similarity measure between two time series, based on Pearson's correlation coefficient, which uses the notion of weighted mean and weighted covariance, where the weights increase monotonically with the time. In the previous chapter, we have also used a weighted similarity measure, between two variables (in this case observation times), that is, two columns of the data matrix. Here, the weighted similarity is between two time series, that is, between two rows of the data matrix.

As pointed out by Caiado et al. [17], a fundamental problem in the clustering of time series is the choice of a relevant metric. For us, two time series are similar to each other, and should therefore fall into the same cluster, if their evolution over time shows similar characteristics. Consider for instance the example in Beringer and Hüllermeier [5], where two stocks both of which continuously increase between 9:00 A.M. and 10:30 A.M. but then started to decrease until 11:30 A.M. are considered similar, no matter what their absolute values are. That is to say that what interests us is not the usual Euclidenan distance between two time series but the distance between their "profiles", which in our case consist in the standardization of the two time series. We will start thus by deriving an expression for this distance. We will

© The Author(s) 2015
J. Pinto da Costa, *Rankings and Preferences*,
SpringerBriefs in Statistics, DOI 10.1007/978-3-662-48344-2_6

change slightly the initial notation from the previous chapter in order to avoid an unnecessary complicated notation.

Let $E = \{X_1, X_2, \ldots, X_n\}$ be a set of n time series each one with p observations and $X_i = (x_{i1}, x_{i2}, \ldots, x_{ip})'$ and $X_l = (x_{l1}, x_{l2}, \ldots, x_{lp})'$ represent the values of two time series which, without loss of generality, started at time 1 and are currently at time p. Our dataset is represented by a $n \times p$ matrix $\mathbf{X}_{n \times p}$ of real numbers whose lines represent the n time series and the columns the observation times; thus, X_i and X_l are two rows of this matrix.

Let us start by standardizing the data but this time, contrary to the previous chapter, standardizing by row instead of by column; that is, taking each time series separately:

$$x_{ij} \leftarrow \frac{x_{ij} - \overline{x}_{i\bullet}}{s_{i\bullet}}, \tag{6.1}$$

where $\overline{x}_{i\bullet} = \frac{1}{p}\sum_{j=1}^{p} x_{ij}$ is the usual average of the values of time series X_i; that is, the average of the values inside the row of the data matrix which corresponds to time series X_i. $s_{i\bullet}^2 = \frac{1}{p}\sum_{j=1}^{p}(x_{ij} - \overline{x}_{i\bullet})^2$ is the variance of time series X_i. The usual squared Euclidean distance between the normalized values of the time series X_i and X_l is

$$\sum_{j=1}^{p}\left(\frac{x_{ij} - \overline{x}_{i\bullet}}{s_{i\bullet}} - \frac{x_{lj} - \overline{x}_{l\bullet}}{s_{l\bullet}}\right)^2$$

$$= \sum_{j=1}^{p}\left\{\frac{(x_{ij} - \overline{x}_{i\bullet})^2}{s_{i\bullet}^2} + \frac{(x_{lj} - \overline{x}_{l\bullet})^2}{s_{l\bullet}^2} - 2\frac{(x_{ij} - \overline{x}_{i\bullet})(x_{lj} - \overline{x}_{l\bullet})}{s_{i\bullet}s_{l\bullet}}\right\}.$$

This equation gives $2p(1-r)$, where r is the Pearson correlation coefficient between the two series X_i and X_l and so we conclude that the squared Euclidean distance between two standardized time series is proportional to $1 - r$.

As is clear from the above expressions, the sample mean and variance give the same importance (weight) to all the values of the time series, namely $\frac{1}{p}$. However, there are situations where this should not be the case; particularly with time series data. It is frequent that with this kind of data the most recent values should be given higher weight, as they are most important for the analysis. Consider for instance again, the situation of the two stocks mentioned above. It is common that investors want to know which stocks are correlated but the recent behavior of the stocks is certainly more important for them then what happened one year ago, let us say. In order to take this into account, we will define now a weighted measure of correlation between two time series. Let us start by defining the weighted moments of mean and variance of time series X_i by

$$\overline{x}_{Pi\bullet} = \sum_{j=1}^{p} w_j x_{ij}, \quad s_{Pi\bullet}^2 = \sum_{j=1}^{p} w_j (x_{ij} - \overline{x}_{i\bullet})^2, \tag{6.2}$$

where the weights w_j are such that $w_j \geq 0$ and $\sum_{j=1}^{p} w_j = 1$. If now we use a weighted Euclidean distance between the weighted standardizations of the time series X_i and X_l we get

$$\sum_{j=1}^{p} w_j \left(\frac{x_{ij} - \bar{x}_{i\bullet}}{s_{Pi\bullet}} - \frac{x_{lj} - \bar{x}_{l\bullet}}{s_{Pl\bullet}} \right)^2 = 2(1 - r_P), \quad \text{where}$$

$$r_P = \frac{\sum_{j=1}^{p} w_j (x_{ij} - \bar{x}_{i\bullet})(x_{lj} - \bar{x}_{l\bullet})}{\sqrt{\sum_{j=1}^{p} w_j (x_{ij} - \bar{x}_{i\bullet})^2} \sqrt{\sum_{j=1}^{p} w_j (x_{lj} - \bar{x}_{l\bullet})^2}} \tag{6.3}$$

is a weighted measure of correlation between the two time series X_i and X_l. Now, instead of using the dissimilarity $d = 1 - r$ we can use $d_1 = 1 - r_P$ to define the distance between the time series. On the other hand, if instead of transformation (6.1) we start by doing the data transformation,

$$x_{ij} \leftarrow \frac{\sqrt{w_j}(x_{ij} - \bar{x}_{i\bullet})}{s_{Pi\bullet}}, \tag{6.4}$$

(similarly for time series X_l) and then we use the usual squared Euclidean distance, the result will be the same.

As in this work we want to give higher importance to the most recent observations, we will use weights like $w_j = j$, $w_j = j^2$, and $w_j = \alpha^j$, for a suitable choice of α (in our applications we use $\alpha = 1.3$). In this work we want to give higher importance to the most recent values but in other situations or for other types of data we might want to prioritize other observations. All that is needed is to choose an appropriate weight function.

The aim of cluster analysis is to find a structure, if it exists, in a dataset, which means to group similar elements in the same cluster and dissimilar elements in different clusters. In our case we want to cluster the n time series in homogeneous clusters. One of the fundamental aspects of cluster analysis is the definition of a proper similarity or dissimilarity index between the elements to be clustered. In our case we choose the indices just described, which are metrics between time series. There are essentially two types of clustering methods: hierarchical and partitional. In order to illustrate the use of weighted clustering in the context of time series, we will use a very well-known partitional method, namely the K-means, with some adaptations to make it able to choose the number of clusters (see [52]).

6.2 Applications

In this section we will apply the weighted clustering in order to analyze a time series dataset that consists of 20 time series with 309 data points, about the Industrial Production (by Market Group) indices in the United States, from January 1977 to September 2002 (source: http://www.economagic.com). This dataset has originated another dataset, the one used in Caiado et al. [17] which contains a specific transformation ($y_{ij} = \log(x_{ij}) - \log(x_{i(j-1)})$) in order to turn on the time series into stationary series.

In Table 6.1, we present the data transformation (DT), the weight function, the number of clusters (K), and the number of series per cluster for the two datasets. In Fig. 6.1, we present the diagram for the partitions obtained with the original Industrial Production indices series, to illustrate our procedure. In (a) we used data transformations corresponding to equations DT = (6.1) and DT = (6.4) with a linear weight and in (b) and (c) we used data transformation DT = (6.4) with quadratic and exponential weights, respectively.

The first observation regarding these results is that the number of clusters has a tendency to reduce when we go from the non-weighted situation (a) to the linear, quadratic, and then exponential weighted cases. It seems that the larger the weight the less clusters we have. However, this conclusion is for this dataset only and we cannot extrapolate. Other experiments are needed and we believe that it is possible that an opposite behavior can be observed with other datasets; it all depends on the structure of the most recent observations of the time series compared to the first. Second, the homogeneity between the initial values of the time series inside each cluster seems to decrease as again we go from the non-weighted situation to the extreme exponential weight case. This behavior was expected as these initial values

Table 6.1 Weighted clustering results for the two datasets

Ind. Prod.	DT	Weight function	K	Series by cluster
Original	1	–	3	16; 3; 1
	2	Linear	3	16; 3; 1
	2	Quadratic	3	17; 2; 1
	2	Exponential	2	18; 2
Stationary	1	–	12	5; 1; 1; 3; 1; 1; 1; 1; 2; 1; 1; 2
	2	Linear or quadratic	13	4; 1; 1; 3; 1; 1; 1; 1; 2; 1; 1; 1; 2
	2	Exponential	8	4; 2; 3; 2; 2; 3; 1; 3

Fig. 6.1 Chronograms of
the original industrial
production indices series

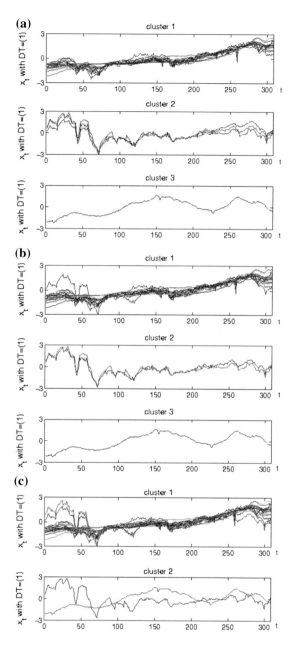

have smaller importance in the weighted cases. As for the last values of the time
series in each cluster, it is difficult to form a conclusion, because on the one hand the
time series should be more and more homogeneous in the last values in the weighted
cases compared to the non-weighted; on the other hand, as in the weighted cases we
have fewer and fewer clusters, the homogeneity inside each cluster decreases.

Appendix

A.1 Maximum Value of the Weighted Distance Function Corresponding to r_W

In Sect. 2.3, we have stated that the maximum value for the distance function used in the weighted rank measure of correlation is obtained when $Q_i = n - R_i + 1$. Here we prove this claim. As in Sect. 2.4, we assume two vectors of ranks, $\boldsymbol{R} = (R_1, \ldots, R_n)$ and $\boldsymbol{Q} = (Q_1, \ldots, Q_n)$.

Proof For the sake of simplicity and without loss of generality we can state this problem as follows. We want to prove that the permutation $(R_1, \ldots, R_n)$ of $(1, \ldots, n)$ that maximizes the expression

$$\sum_{i=1}^{n}(i - R_i)^2\big((n - i + 1) + (n - R_i + 1)\big) = \sum_{i=1}^{n}(i - R_i)^2\big(2(n+1) - i - R_i\big) \quad \text{(A.1)}$$

is the permutation $(n, \ldots, 1)$; that is, $R_i = n - i + 1$. In other words, we assume that $Q_i = i$.

Suppose that this is not the optimal permutation. Let us then assume that the optimal permutation is $(R'_1, \ldots, R'_n)$. This means that there exist at least two integers, ℓ and m, smaller than or equal to n, such that $R'_\ell \neq R_\ell$ and $R'_m \neq R_m$.

Let us then denote by $\ell = \min_{i=1,\ldots,n}\big\{i : R'_i \neq n - i + 1\big\}$, that is, ℓ is the first integer for which $R'_\ell \neq n - \ell + 1$. It is clear that $R'_\ell < R_\ell = n - \ell + 1$. Now let us consider m such that $R'_m = R_\ell = n - \ell + 1$. We, thus, have the following situation:

1	2	...	$\ell - 1$	ℓ	...	m	...	n
$\boldsymbol{R}$ n	$n-1$	...	$n-\ell+2$	$n-\ell+1$	...	$n-m+1$	...	1
$\boldsymbol{R'}$ n	$n-1$	...	$n-\ell+2$	R'_ℓ	...	$n-\ell+1$	...	R'_n

We will now demonstrate that if we swap R'_ℓ with R'_m in permutation $\boldsymbol{R'}$ we obtain a 'better' partition, which is absurd, since $\boldsymbol{R'}$ is the optimum permutation by hypothesis.

© The Author(s) 2015
J. Pinto da Costa, *Rankings and Preferences*,
SpringerBriefs in Statistics, DOI 10.1007/978-3-662-48344-2

If we swap R'_ℓ with R'_m then R_ℓ will be placed in the position of R'_ℓ and R'_ℓ will be in the position of R'_m. The value of sum (A.1) after the change will differ by:

$$(\ell - R_\ell)^2(n - \ell + 1 + n - R_\ell + 1) + (m - R'_\ell)^2(n - m + 1 + n - R'_\ell + 1)$$
$$- (\ell - R'_\ell)^2(n - \ell + 1 + n - R'_\ell + 1) + (m - R_\ell)^2(n - m + 1 + n - R_\ell + 1)$$
$$= -(m - \ell)(R'_\ell - R_\ell)(4n + 4 - \ell - m - R_\ell - R'_\ell) > 0$$

because $m - \ell > 0$, $R'_\ell < R_\ell$ and $\ell, m, R_\ell, R'_\ell \le n$.

We thus prove that the value of sum (A.1) enlarges, which is absurd given that by hypothesis $\boldsymbol{R'}$ is the optimal partition. Since this hypothesis is false, the best permutation is $\boldsymbol{R}$, that is $(n, \ldots, 1)$.

The maximum value of the weighted distance between two rankings is therefore $\sum_{i=1}^{n} W_i^2 = \sum_{i=1}^{n}(2R_i - n - 1)^2(n + 1) = (n^4 + n^3 - n^2 - n)/3$.

A.2 Maximum Value of the Weighted Distance Function Corresponding to r_{W2}

Here we show that the maximum value for the distance function $\sum_{i=1}^{n} W_2 D_i^2$ used in Sect. 3 is obtained when $Q_i = n + 1 - R_i$.

Theorem 3 *The maximum value for* $\sum_{i=1}^{n}(R_i - Q_i)^2(2n + 2 - R_i - Q_i)^2$ *is* $\frac{n(n-1)(n+1)^3}{3}$ *and is obtained when* $Q_i = n + 1 - R_i$.

Proof we consider two vectors of ranks $R = (R_1, \ldots, R_n)$ and $Q = (Q_1, \ldots, Q_n)$. Without loss of generality we assume $Q_i = i$ and $R_i = n+1-i, i = 1, \ldots, n$. If we suppose that the permutation $R = (n, \ldots, 1)$ is not the permutation that maximizes $\sum_{i=1}^{n}(R_i - Q_i)^2(2n + 2 - R_i - Q_i)^2$ when we evaluate with the natural order $Q = (1, \ldots, n)$, then there is another ranking $\grave{R} = (\grave{R}_1, \ldots, \grave{R}_n)$, different from R, that is a optimal permutation. Thus, there are at least two positions, say l and m, in vectors R and $\grave{R}$, such that $R_l \ne \grave{R}_l$ and $R_m \ne \grave{R}_m$. Let l be the first integer for which $\grave{R}_l \ne n + 1 - l$. We note that $\grave{R}_l < R_l = n - l + 1$. We consider m such that $\grave{R}_m = R_l = n - l + 1$. Analogously to our proof in A.1 we have the following situation:

Q	1	2	...	$l-1$	l	...	m	...	n
R	n	$n-1$	...	$n+2-l$	$n+1-l$	...	$n+1-m$	...	1
$\grave{R}$	n	$n-1$	...	$n+2-l$	$\grave{R}_l$	...	$n+1-l$	...	$\grave{R}_n$

If we swap $\grave{R}_l$ with $\grave{R}_m$ in permutation $\grave{R}$ we obtain a better permutation, since the value of $\sum_{i=1}^{n}(R_i - Q_i)^2(2n + 2 - R_i - Q_i)^2$ after the swap will differ by:

$$(l - R_l)^2 (2n + 2 - l - R_l)^2 + (m - \grave{R}_l)^2 (2n + 2 - m - \grave{R}_l)^2$$
$$- (l - \grave{R}_l)^2 (2n + 2 - l - \grave{R}_l)^2 + (m - R_l)^2 (2n + 2 - m - R_l)^2$$
$$= (m - l)(R_l - \grave{R}_l) \left[m(2\grave{R}_l - 4 - 4n) + \grave{R}_l(2l - 4 - 4n) + r_l(2m - 4 - 4n) \right.$$
$$\left. + l(2r_l - 4 - 4n) + 8(n + 1)^2 \right] > 0.$$

This is absurd because by hypothesis $\grave{R}$ is the optimal permutation. Thus, the optimal permutation can only be R.

We note that the last product above is positive because $m - l > 0$, $R_l - \grave{R}_l > 0$; $m, l, r_l, \grave{R}_l \leq n$ and

$$m(2\grave{R}_l - 4 - 4n) + \grave{R}_l(2l - 4 - 4n) + R_l(2m - 4 - 4n) + l(2R_l - 4 - 4n) + 8(n + 1)^2$$
$$= 8(n + 1)^2 - 4(n + 1)(m + l + \grave{R}_l + R_l) + 2(m + l)(\grave{R}_l + R_l) > 0.$$

In order to prove the last inequality, suppose that there exists $m, l, r_l, \grave{r}_l \in \{1, \dots, n\}$ such that

$$8(n + 1)^2 - 4(n + 1)(m + l + \grave{R}_l + R_l) + 2(m + l)(\grave{R}_l + R_l) = 0.$$

Then, we have $m + l = 2n + 2$ or $\grave{r}_l + r_l = 2n + 2$, which is absurd because $m, l, r_l, \grave{r}_l \leq n$. If we suppose that,

$$8(n + 1)^2 - 4(n + 1)(m + l + \grave{R}_l + r_l) + 2(m + l)(\grave{R}_l + r_l) < 0,$$

then $min\left\{ \frac{m+l}{2}, \frac{\grave{R}_l + R_l}{2} \right\} < n + 1 < max \left\{ \frac{m+l}{2}, \frac{\grave{R}_l + R_l}{2} \right\}$, which is absurd because $m, l, R_l, \grave{R}_l \leq n$. Therefore, we have

$$8(n + 1)^2 - 4(n + 1)(m + l + \grave{R}_l + R_l) + 2(m + l)(\grave{R}_l + R_l) > 0.$$

A.3 Mean and Variance of r_W Under the Null Hypothesis

Here we prove the theorem from Sect. 2.4.

Proof We start by rewriting r_W as a linear combination of linear rank statistics:

$$\sum_{i=1}^{n} (i - R_i^*)^2 (2(n + 1) - i - R_i^*)$$

$$= 4(n + 1) \sum_{i=1}^{n} i^2 - 2 \sum_{i=1}^{n} i^3 + \sum_{i=1}^{n} i^2 R_i^* + \sum_{i=1}^{n} i R_i^{*2} - 4(n + 1) \sum_{i=1}^{n} i R_i^*$$

The term $4(n+1)\sum_{i=1}^{n} i^2 - 2\sum_{i=1}^{n} i^3$ does not depend on $\boldsymbol{R}^*$ and so is a constant, that we denote by C. Let,

$$S_n^{(11)} = \sum_{i=1}^{n} i\, R_i^*, \quad S_n^{(12)} = \sum_{i=1}^{n} i\, R_i^{*2} \quad \text{and} \quad S_n^{(21)} = \sum_{i=1}^{n} i^2 R_i^*.$$

The distribution of r_W under H_0 is the same as that of

$$1 - \frac{6C}{n(n^3+n^2-n-1)} + \frac{24(n+1)}{n(n^3+n^2-n-1)} S_n^{(11)}$$
$$- \frac{6}{n(n^3+n^2-n-1)} S_n^{(12)} - \frac{6}{n(n^3+n^2-n-1)} S_n^{(21)} \qquad (A.2)$$

Using (2.3), we get,

$$E(S_n^{(11)}) = n\frac{\sum_{i=1}^{n} i \sum_{i=1}^{n} i}{n} = \frac{n(n+1)^2}{4},$$
$$E(S_n^{(12)}) = n\frac{\sum_{i=1}^{n} i \sum_{i=1}^{n} i^2}{n} = \frac{n(n+1)}{2}\frac{n(n+1)(2n+1)}{6n} = \frac{n(n+1)^2(2n+1)}{12}$$
$$E(S_n^{(21)}) = n\frac{\sum_{i=1}^{n} i^2 \sum_{i=1}^{n} i}{n} = \frac{n(n+1)}{2}\frac{n(n+1)(2n+1)}{6n} = \frac{n(n+1)^2(2n+1)}{12}$$

and so:

$$E(r_W) = 1 - \frac{6C - 6(n+1)^3 n + n(n+1)^2(2n+1)}{n(n^3+n^2-n-1)} = 0.$$

We see therefore that if the two vectors of ranks are independent, the expected value of the weighted rank measure of correlation is 0, which is a desirable property. Let us now find an expression for the variance of r_W under H_0:

$$\text{var}(r_W) = \left(\frac{6}{n(n^3+n^2-n-1)}\right)^2 \text{var}\left(4(n+1)S_n^{(11)} - S_n^{(12)} - S_n^{(21)}\right)$$
$$= \left(\frac{6}{n(n^3+n^2-n-1)}\right)^2 \left(16(n+1)^2\text{var}(S_n^{(11)}) + \text{var}(S_n^{(12)}) + \text{var}(S_n^{(21)})\right.$$
$$\left. - 8(n+1)\text{cov}(S_n^{(11)}, S_n^{(12)}) - 8(n+1)\text{cov}(S_n^{(11)}, S_n^{(21)}) + 2\text{cov}(S_n^{(12)}, S_n^{(21)})\right)$$
$$\hspace{10cm} (A.3)$$

To find the variance of $S_n^{(11)} = \sum_{i=1}^{n} i\, R_i^*$, note that $S_n^{(11)}$ has the expression in (2.2) if $c(i) = i$ and $a(i) = i$. Therefore, by (2.3),

$$\text{var}(S_n^{(11)}) = \frac{1}{n-1}\left(\sum_{i=1}^{n} i^2 - n\frac{(n+1)^2}{4}\right)\left(\sum_{i=1}^{n} i^2 - n\frac{(n+1)^2}{4}\right)$$

$$= \frac{n^2(n+1)^2(n-1)}{144}$$

For $S_n^{(12)} = \sum_{i=1}^{n} i R_i^{*2}$, as $c(i) = i$ and $a(i) = i^2$, the variance becomes

$$\text{var}(S_n^{(12)}) = \frac{1}{n-1}\left(\sum_{i=1}^{n} i^2 - n\frac{(n+1)^2}{4}\right)\left(\sum_{i=1}^{n} i^4 - n\frac{(n+1)^2(2n+1)^2}{36}\right)$$

$$= \frac{n^2(n+1)^2}{2160}(16n^3 + 14n^2 - 19n - 11)$$

On the other hand, as $S_n^{(21)} = \sum_{i=1}^{n} i^2 R_i^*$, we have $\text{var}(S_n^{(21)}) = \text{var}(S_n^{(12)})$. We also need to find the covariance between two linear rank statistics. In [79, Chap. 8] if

$$S' = \sum_{i=1}^{n} c'(i)a'(R_i^*),$$

is another linear rank statistic then, under H_0,

$$\text{cov}(S, S') = (n-1)s_{cc'}s_{aa'}$$

and so,

$$\text{cov}(S_n^{(11)}, S_n^{(12)}) = \text{cov}(S_n^{(11)}, S_n^{(21)}) = \frac{1}{144}(n^4 + 2n^3 - 2n - 1)n^2$$

Similarly,

$$\text{cov}(S_n^{(12)}, S_n^{(21)}) = \frac{1}{144}(n^5 + 3n^4 + 2n^3 - 2n^2 - 3n - 1)n^2$$

Finally, substituting all these results in (A.3), we get the variance of r_W under the null hypothesis of independence between the two vectors of ranks:

$$\text{var}(r_W) = \frac{31n^2 + 60n + 26}{30(n^3 + n^2 - n - 1)}$$

With this notation, the expression (A.2) for r_W can be written in the form:

$$
r_W = \frac{1}{n(n^3 + n^2 - n - 1)} \Bigg(n(n^3 + n^2 - n - 1) - 24\frac{(n+1)^2 n(2n+1)}{6}
$$

$$
+ 12\frac{n^2(n+1)^2}{4} + 24(n+1)\big(S_n^{(11)} - \mathrm{E}(S_n^{(11)})\big)
$$

$$
+ 24\frac{(n+1)^3 n}{4} - 6\big(S_n^{(12)} - \mathrm{E}(S_n^{(12)})\big)
$$

$$
- 6\big(S_n^{(21)} - \mathrm{E}(S_n^{(21)})\big) - n(n+1)^2(2n+1) \Bigg)
$$

But

$$
n(n^3 + n^2 - n - 1) - 4(n+1)^2 n(2n+1) + 3n^2(n+1)^2
$$
$$
+ 6(n+1)^3 n - n(n+1)^2(2n+1) = 0,
$$

and so

$$
r_W = \frac{1}{n(n^3 + n^2 - n - 1)} \Bigg(24(n+1)\big(S_n^{(11)} - \mathrm{E}(S_n^{(11)})\big)
$$

$$
- 6\big(S_n^{(12)} - \mathrm{E}(S_n^{(12)})\big) - 6\big(S_n^{(21)} - \mathrm{E}(S_n^{(21)})\big) \Bigg)
$$

A.4 Table of Critical Values for r_W

In the following table we present the most important quantiles for r_W under the null hypothesis that the two vectors of ranks are independent (Table A.1).

A.5 Asymptotic Normality of Nonparametric Statistics

We present in this Appendix Theorem 2.1 of Ruymgaart, Shorack and Van Zwet, 1972 (see [84]) as is the fundamental tool used in the proof of our Theorem 2.1. We start by introducing some notation. Let $(X_1, Y_1), \ldots, (X_n, Y_n)$ be a random sample from a continuous bivariate distribution function $H(x, y)$ (bivariate empirical distribution function is denoted by H_n) having marginal distribution functions $F(x)$ and $G(y)$ and empirical distribution functions F_n and G_n, respectively. The rank of X_i is denoted by R_i and the rank of Y_i by Q_i. Let $T_n = \frac{1}{n}\sum_{i=1}^{n} a_n(R_i)b_n(Q_i)$, where $a_n(i), b_n(i)$ are real numbers for $i = 1, \ldots, n$. The standardization of T_n can be written as

$$
\sqrt{n}(T_n - \mu) = \sqrt{n}\left[\int\int J_n(F_n) K_n(G_n)\, dH_n - \mu \right],
$$

Table A.1 Critical values for r_W

n	Confidence level (%)							
	0.5	1	2.5	5	95	97.5	99	99.5
3	–	–	–	–	1.0000	1.0000	1.0000	1.0000
4	–	–	–	-1.0000	0.8800	1.0000	1.0000	1.0000
5	–	-1.0000	-1.0000	-0.9000	0.8000	0.8833	0.9500	1.0000
6	-1.0000	-0.9429	-0.8286	-0.7714	0.7388	0.8122	0.9020	0.9429
7	-0.8973	-0.8571	-0.7768	-0.6875	0.6830	0.7812	0.8571	0.8973
8	-0.8624	-0.8095	-0.7196	-0.6323	0.6402	0.7275	0.8148	0.8624
9	-0.8167	-0.7667	-0.6800	-0.5917	0.5967	0.6883	0.7750	0.8233
10	-0.7807	-0.7311	-0.6441	-0.5559	0.5614	0.6518	0.7399	0.7917
11	-0.7508	-0.6992	-0.6121	-0.5280	0.5326	0.6197	0.7091	0.7614
12	-0.7230	-0.6708	-0.5853	-0.5035	0.5073	0.5922	0.6810	0.7337
13	-0.6978	-0.6460	-0.5616	-0.4819	0.4855	0.5675	0.6550	0.7084
14	-0.6750	-0.6234	-0.5405	-0.4629	0.4664	0.5461	0.6319	0.6850
15	-0.6534	-0.6023	-0.5210	-0.4454	0.4497	0.5279	0.6111	0.6645
16	-0.6353	-0.5850	-0.5056	-0.4314	0.4342	0.5091	0.5911	0.6432
17	-0.6177	-0.5677	-0.4893	-0.4170	0.4193	0.4931	0.5738	0.6252
18	-0.6012	-0.5525	-0.4758	-0.4051	0.4064	0.4784	0.5583	0.6092
19	-0.5854	-0.5374	-0.4621	-0.3935	0.3950	0.4650	0.5433	0.5935
20	-0.5725	-0.5247	-0.4505	-0.3837	0.3850	0.4539	0.5306	0.5797
25	-0.5135	-0.4693	-0.4012	-0.3407	0.3423	0.4045	0.4744	0.5203
30	-0.4720	-0.4296	-0.3660	-0.3103	0.3112	0.3679	0.4316	0.4740
40	-0.4029	-0.3668	-0.3113	-0.2629	0.2650	0.3156	0.3721	0.4095
50	-0.3590	-0.3273	-0.2786	-0.2356	0.2361	0.2807	0.3316	0.3658

For n up to 14 the values were obtained by computing all the permutations. For other values they are approximated using a random sample of one million rankings. For $n > 50$, the quantiles for the standardized measure are approximated by the Standard Normal: $\left(\frac{30(n^3+n^2-n-1)}{31n^2+60n+26}\right)^{1/2} r_W \overset{d}{\approx} N(0,1)$

where $J_n(s) = a_n(i)$, $K_n(s) = b_n(i)$, for $i = 1, \ldots, n$ such that $\frac{(i-1)}{n} < s \le \frac{i}{n}$; $\mu = \int\int J(F)K(G)dH$. The functions J and K can be thought of as limits of the score functions J_n and K_n. $\mathscr{H}$ denote the class of all continuous bivariate distribution functions H.

Assumption 2.1 (Ruymgaart, Shorack and Van Zwet 1972) The functions J and K are continuous on $(0, 1)$; each is differentiable except at most at a finite number of points, and in the open intervals between these points the derivatives are continuous. The functions J_n, K_n, J, K satisfy $|J_n| \le Dr^a$, $|K_n| \le Dr^a$ and $\left|J^{(i)}\right| \le Dr^{a+i}$ and $\left|K^{(i)}\right| \le Dr^{b+i}$ for $i = 0, 1$. Here D is a positive constant, $a = \frac{\left(\frac{1}{2}-\delta\right)}{p}$, $b = \frac{\left(\frac{1}{2}-\delta\right)}{q}$ for some $0 < \delta < \frac{1}{2}$ and some $p, q > 1$ with $\frac{1}{p} + \frac{1}{q} = 1$.

Assumption 2.3 b (Ruymgaart, Shorack and Van Zwet 1972) $B_{0n}^* = \sqrt{n} \int \int$ $\left[J_n(F_n)K_n(G_n) - J(F_n^*)K(G_n^*) \right] dH_n \underset{p}{\rightarrow} 0$ (converge in probability to zero) as

$n \to \infty$ where $F_n^* = \left[\frac{n}{n+1} \right] F_n$ and $G_n^* = \left[\frac{n}{n+1} \right] G_n$.

Theorem 2.1 of Ruymgaart, Shorack and Van Zwet 1972 (see [84])
If H is in $\mathscr{H}$ and if Assumptions 2.1 and 2.3 b are satisfied, then $\sqrt{n}(T_n - \mu) \underset{d}{\rightarrow} N(0, \sigma^2)$ (converge in distribution) as $n \to \infty$, where μ and σ^2 are finite and are given by $\mu = \int \int J(F)K(G)dH$ (expression 1.3 in [84]) and

$$\sigma^2 = Var \left[J(F(X))K(G(Y)) + \int \int (\phi_X - F)J'(F)K(G)dH \right.$$
$$\left. + \int \int (\phi_Y - G)J(F)K'(G)dH \right]$$

(expression 3.10 in [84]) with $\phi_{X_i}(x) = 0$ if $x < X_i$ and $\phi_{X_i}(x) = 1$ if $x \geq X_i$.

A.6 A_{1in} has a Finite Absolute Moment of Order Greater than 2

We show here that there exist $\delta_0 > 0$ and $\delta_0 < \delta = \frac{1}{4}$ such that $E|A_{1in}|^{2+\delta_0}$ is bounded. Using Assumption 2.1 in the Appendix above we can prove that

$$\int \int |J(F(X_i), G(Y_i))|^{2+\delta_0} dH \leq D \int \int |r(F)|^{a(2+\delta_0)} |r(G)|^{b(2+\delta_0)} dH.$$

By using now Hölder's Inequality this quantity is

$$\leq D \frac{1}{n} \sum_{i=1}^{n} \left\{ r^{(2+\delta_0)(\delta-\frac{1}{2})} \left(\frac{i}{n+1} \right) \right\}^{\frac{1}{p_0}} \left\{ \frac{1}{n} \sum_{i=1}^{n} r^{(2+\delta_0)(\delta-\frac{1}{2})} \left(\frac{i}{n+1} \right) \right\}^{\frac{1}{q_0}}$$

$$= \frac{D}{n} \sum r^{(2+\delta_0)(\delta-\frac{1}{2})} \left(\frac{i}{n+1} \right)$$

$$\leq D \int_0^1 \frac{1}{(u(1-u))^{(2+\delta_0)(\frac{1}{2}-\delta)}} du$$

that is finite for $0 < \delta_0 < \delta = \frac{1}{4}$.

A.7 Calculation of the Alternative Expression for r_{W2}

Theorem 4 $r_{W2} = \frac{1}{2}\frac{V_{R'}+V_{Q'}-D_{W2n}}{\sqrt{V_{R'}}\sqrt{V_{Q'}}}$, *where $V_{R'}$ and $V_{Q'}$ are the variances of the transformed rankings R' and Q', respectively, and D_{W2n} (3.7) is the weighted distance between the two rankings.*

Proof First, we observe that $\overline{R'} = \frac{1}{n}\sum_{i=1}^{n}(R_i(2n+2-R_i)) = \frac{(n+1)(4n+5)}{6} = \gamma(n)$ and similarly for $\overline{Q'}$. We define $V_{R'}$, $V_{Q'}$ and D_{W2n} as before. Recall the quantities:

$$V_{R'} = \frac{1}{n}\sum_{i=1}^{n}\left[R_i(2n+2-R_i)-\gamma(n)\right]^2,$$

$$V_{Q'} = \frac{1}{n}\sum_{i=1}^{n}\left[Q_i(2n+2-Q_i)-\gamma(n)\right]^2$$

and

$$D_{W2n} = \frac{1}{n}\sum_{i=1}^{n}(R_i-Q_i)^2(2n+2-R_i-Q_i)^2.$$

Now, we consider Pearson's correlation coefficient of the transformed rankings R' and Q',

$$r_{W2} = \frac{\sum_{i=1}^{n}\left[(R_i(2n+2-R_i)-\gamma(n))\cdot(Q_i(2n+2-Q_i)-\gamma(n))\right]}{\sqrt{\sum_{i=1}^{n}(R_i(2n+2-R_i)-\gamma(n))^2}\sqrt{\sum_{i=1}^{n}(Q_i(2n+2-Q_i)-\gamma(n))^2}}.$$

It is convenient to note that

$$2\cdot\sum_{i=1}^{n}\left[(R_i(2n+2-R_i)-\gamma(n))\cdot(Q_i(2n+2-Q_i)-\gamma(n))\right]$$

$$=\sum_{i=1}^{n}(R_i(2n+2-R_i)-\gamma(n))^2+\sum_{i=1}^{n}(Q_i(2n+2-Q_i)-\gamma(n))^2$$

$$-\sum_{i=1}^{n}(R_i(2n+2-R_i)-Q_i(2n+2-Q_i))^2$$

and

$$\sum_{i=1}^{n} (R_i (2n + 2 - R_i) - Q_i (2n + 2 - Q_i))^2$$

$$= \sum_{i=1}^{n} (R_i - Q_i)^2 (2n + 2 - R_i - Q_i)^2 = n D_{W2n}.$$

Therefore, $r_{W2} = \frac{1}{2} \frac{V_{R'} + V_{Q'} - D_{W2n}}{\sqrt{V_{R'}} \sqrt{V_{Q'}}}$.

For untied ranking the quantities $V_{R'}$ and $V_{Q'}$ are

$$V_{Q'} = V_{R'} = \frac{g(n)}{180n}$$

and it follows that r_{W2} can be written as

$$r_{W2} = 1 - \frac{90n D_{W2n}}{g(n)}.$$

A.8 Appendix—Computation of the Principal Components in the Case of More Variables than Observations

A.8.1 Computation of the Unweighted Principal Components

Let us start by denoting by $\mathbb{X}$ the data matrix with n rows, corresponding to the n samples, and p columns, corresponding to the p variables. In the usual PCA, we must find the $p \times p$ matrix of Pearson's correlation coefficients. To do so, we start by standardising the data as

$$x_{ij} \leftarrow \frac{x_{ij} - \bar{x}_j}{s_j \sqrt{n}}, \tag{A.4}$$

where $\bar{x}_j$ is the mean value of variable j and $s_j^2 = \frac{1}{n} \sum_{l=1}^{n} (x_{lj} - \bar{x}_j)^2$ the corresponding sample variance. The matrix of Pearson's correlations is then $\mathbb{X}^T \mathbb{X}$. The analysis that follows consists in finding the eigenvectors and eigenvalues of this matrix. However, because if we have a relatively large number of variables and much lesser samples, this matrix will have a huge dimension and will not have full rank. It is complicated and very time consuming to diagonalise such a matrix and what is usually done consists in finding the eigenvectors and eigenvalues of the matrix $\mathbb{X}\mathbb{X}^T$ instead, and from these find the ones we want. If x is an unit eigenvector of $\mathbb{X}\mathbb{X}^T$ and λ the corresponding eigenvalue, then

$$\mathbb{X}\mathbb{X}^T x = \lambda x.$$

Pre-multiplying this equation by $\mathbb{X}^T$ gives

$$\mathbb{X}^T \mathbb{X} \mathbb{X}^T x = \lambda \mathbb{X}^T x,$$

which means that $\mathbb{X}^T x$ is an eigenvector of $\mathbb{X}^T \mathbb{X}$ with the same eigenvalue λ. To normalise this eigenvector, let us find its norm as

$$||\mathbb{X}^T x||^2 = (\mathbb{X}^T x)^T \mathbb{X}^T x = x^T \mathbb{X} \mathbb{X}^T x = x^T \lambda x = \lambda,$$

because the norm of x is 1. Hence, $||\mathbb{X}^T x|| = \sqrt{\lambda}$. Therefore, we conclude that if x is an unit eigenvector of $\mathbb{X} \mathbb{X}^T$ and λ the corresponding eigenvalue, then $\frac{1}{\sqrt{\lambda}} \mathbb{X}^T x$ is a unit eigenvector of the matrix $\mathbb{X}^T \mathbb{X}$ with the same eigenvalue λ. This is a very useful result because it allows us to find the eigenvectors of a huge matrix, $\mathbb{X}^T \mathbb{X}$, by diagonalising a much smaller matrix, $\mathbb{X} \mathbb{X}^T$.

A.8.2 Computation of the Weighted Principal Components

To compute the weighted principal components, that is, using the correlation coefficient r_{W2}, we start by transforming our data according to equation (4.2). Then, similarly to the previous subsection, we standardise the transformed data as

$$R'_{ij} \leftarrow \frac{R'_{ij} - \overline{R'}_j}{S_{Rj} \sqrt{n}}, \tag{A.5}$$

where $\overline{R'}_j$ is the mean value of the weighted ranks corresponding to variable j and $S_{Rj}^2 = \frac{1}{n} \sum_{l=1}^{n} (R'_{lj} - \overline{R'}_j)^2$ the corresponding sample variance. Hence, if $\mathbb{X}'$ represents the data matrix corresponding to these transformations, the matrix of weighted correlation coefficients (r_{W2}) is $\mathbb{X}'^T \mathbb{X}'$. As before, if this is a huge matrix, in order to obtain its diagonalisation we proceed exactly as for the unweighted case, diagonalising first $\mathbb{X}' \mathbb{X}'^T$. Hence, if x is an unit eigenvector of $\mathbb{X}' \mathbb{X}'^T$ and λ the corresponding eigenvalue, then $\frac{1}{\sqrt{\lambda}} \mathbb{X}'^T x$ is a unit eigenvector of the matrix $\mathbb{X}'^T \mathbb{X}'$ with the same eigenvalue λ.

References

1. Alcock, R. J., & Manolopoulos, Y. (1999). Time-series similarity queries employing a feature-based approach. In *Proceeding of the 7th Hellenic Conference on Informatics, Greece*.
2. Ambroise, C., & McLachlan, G. J. (2002). Selection bias in gene extraction on the basis of microarray gene-expression data. In *Proceedings of the national academy of sciences* (vol. 99, pp. 6562–6566).
3. Badcock, J., Jonathan, P., Bailey, T. C., & Krzanowski, W. J. (2004). Two projection methods for use in the analysis of multivariate process data with an illustration in petrochemical production. *Technometrics, 46*, 392–403.
4. Baeza-Yates, R., & Ribeiro-Neto, B. (1999). *Modern information retrieval*. New York: Addison Wesley.
5. Beringer, J., & Hüllermeier, E. (2006). Online clustering of parallel data streams. *Data and Knowledge Engineering, 58*(2), 107–204.
6. Bicciato, S., Luchini, A., & Di Bello, C. (2003). PCA disjoint models for multiclass cancer analysis using gene expression data. *Bioinformatics, 19*, 571–578.
7. Bhuchongkul, S. (1964). A class of nonparametric tests for independence in bivariate populations. *Annals of Mathematical Statistics, 35*, 138–149.
8. Billingsley, P. (1978). Probability and measure. *Probability and mathematical statistics*. New York: Wiley.
9. Bleichrodt, H., & Johannesson, M. (1997). Standard gamble, time trade-off and rating scale: Experimental results on the ranking properties of QALYs. *Journal of Health Economics, 16*, 155–175.
10. Blest, D. (2000). Rank correlation—An alternative measure. *Australian and New Zealand Journal of Statistics, 42*(1), 101–111.
11. Brazdil, P., & Soares, C. (2000). A comparison of ranking methods for classification algorithm selection. In R. L. Mántaras & E. Plaza (Eds.), *Machine learning: Proceedings of the 11th european conference on machine learning ECML2000* (pp. 63–74). Springer.
12. Brazdil, P., Soares, C., & Pinto da Costa, J. (2003). Ranking learning algorithms: Using IBL and meta-learning on accuracy and time results. *Machine Learning, 50*(3), 251–277.
13. Brazma, A., & Vilo, J. (2000). Gene expression data analysis. *Federation of European Biochemical Societies (FEBS) Letters, 480*, 17–24.
14. Breese, J., Heckerman, D., & Kadie, C. (1998). Empirical analysis of predictive algorithms for collaborative filtering. In *Proceedings of the fourteenth conference on uncertainty in artificial intelligence* (pp. 43–52). Morgan Kaufmann.
15. Breiman, L., Friedman, J. H., Olshen, A., & Stone, C. J. (1984). *Classification and regression trees*. Belmont: Wadsworth.
16. Burges, C. J. C. (1998). A tutorial on support vector machines for pattern recognition. *Data Mining, 2*, 121–167.

17. Caiado, J., Crato, N., & Peña, D. (2006). A periodogram-based metric for time series classification. *Computational Statistics and Data Analysis, 50*(10), 2668–2684.
18. Callan, J., Connel, M., & Du, A. (1999). Automatic discovery of language models for text databases. In A. Delis, C. Faloutsos & S. Ghandeharizadeh (Eds.), *Proceedings of the 1999 ACM SIGMOD international conference on management of data* (pp. 479–490). ACM.
19. Chernoff, H., & Savage, I. R. (1958). Asymptotic normality and efficiency of certain nonparametric test statistics. *Annals of Mathematical Statistics, 29*, 972–994.
20. Dabney, A. R. (2005). Classification of microarray to nearest centroids. *Bioinformatics, 21*(22), 4148–4154.
21. Daniel, W. (1995). *Biostatistics: A foundation for analysis in the health sciences.* Wiley series in probability and mathematical statistics—Applied, Singapore.
22. Megreditchian, Der. (1988). *Le traitement statistique des données multidimensionnelles, Tome I.* Ecola National de la Météorologie, Paris
23. Dudoit, S., Fridlyand, J., & Speed, T. P. (2002). Comparison of discrimination methods for the classification of tumors using gene expression data. *Journal of the American Statistical Association, 97*, 77–87.
24. Ewens, W.J. and Grant, G.R. (2005) *Statistical methods in bioinformatics—An introduction* (2nd ed.). New York: Springer.
25. Faber, J., Krivtsov, A. V., Stubbs, M. C., Wright, R., Davis, T. N., van den Heuvel-Eibrink, M., et al. (2009). HOXA9 is required for survival in human MLL-rearranged acute leukemias. *Blood, 113*(11), 2375–2385.
26. Fisher, R. (1936). The use of multiple measurements in taxonomic problems. *Annals of Eugenics, 7*, 179–188.
27. Gaißer, S. C. (2010). *Statistics for copula-based measures of multivariate association; theory and applications to financial data.* Ph.D. Thesis, University of Cologne.
28. Genest, C., & Plante, J.-F. (2003). On Blest's measure of rank correlation. *The Canadian Journal of Statistics, 31*, 35–52.
29. Genest, C., & Plante, J.-F. (2007). Letter to the editor. *Australian and New Zealand Journal of Statistics, 49*.
30. Gentleman, R., Carey, V. J., Huber, W., Irizarry, R. A., & Dudoit, S. (Eds.). (2005). *Bioinformatics and computational biology solutions using R and Bioconductor.* New York: Springer.
31. Geurts, P. (2002). *Contributions to decision tree induction: Bias/variance tradeoff and time series classification.* Ph.D. thesis, University of Liège, Belgium.
32. Girolami, M., & Breitling, R. (2004). Biologically valid linear factor models of gene expression. *Bioinformatics, 20*, 3021–3033.
33. Harter, S., & Hert, C. (1997). Evaluation of information retrieval systems: Approaches, issues, and methods. *Annual Review of Information Science and Technology (ARIST), 32*, 3–94.
34. Hastie, T., Tibshirani, R., & Friedman, J. (2002). *The elements of statistical learning.* New York: Springer.
35. Hellström, T. (2001). Optimizing the sharpe ratio for a rank based trading system. In P. Brazdil & A. Jorge (Eds.), *LNAI 2258: Proceedings of the 10th Portuguese conference on artificial intelligence* (pp. 130–141). Springer.
36. Hotelling, H. (1935). The most predictable criterion. *Journal of Educational Psychology, 26*, 139–143.
37. Hotelling, H. (1936). Relations between two sets of variates. *Biometrika, 28*, 321–377.
38. Hubert, M., & Engelen, S. (2004). Robust PCA and classification in biosciences. *Bioinformatics, 20*, 1728–1736.
39. Jagadeeswaran, R., Surawska, H., Krishnaswamy, S., Janamanchi, V., Mackinnon, A. C., Seiwert, T. Y., et al. (2008). Paxillin is a target for somatic mutations in lung cancer: implications for cell growth and invasion. *Cancer Research, 68*(1), 132–142.
40. Järvelin, K., & Kekäläinen, J. (2000). IR evaluation methods for retrieving highly relevant documents. In N. Belkin, P. Ingwersen & M.-K. Leong (Eds.), *Proceedings of the 23th annual international ACM SIGIR conference on research and development in information retrieval (ACM SIGIR '00)* (pp. 41–48). ACM Press.

41. Jansen, J. J., Hoefsloot, H. C., Boelens, H. F., van der Greef, J., & Smilde, A. K. (2004). Analysis of longitudinal metabolomics data. *Bioinformatics, 20*, 2438–2446.
42. Jolliffe, T. (2002). *Principal component analysis* (2nd ed.). New York: Springer.
43. Katase, N., Gunduz, M., Beder, L., Gunduz, E., Lefeuvre, M., Hatipoglu, O. F., et al. (2008). Deletion at dickkopf (dkk)-3 locus (11p15.2) is related with lower lymph node metastasis and better prognosis in head and neck squamous cell carcinomas. *Oncology Research, 17*(6), 273–282.
44. Keller, J., Paterson, I., & Berrer, H. (2000). An integrated concept for multi-criteria ranking of data-mining algorithms. In J. Keller, & C. Giraud-Carrier (Eds.), *Meta-learning: Building automatic advice strategies for model selection and method combination.*
45. Kendall, M. G. (1962). *Rank correlation methods.* London: Charles Griffin & Company Limited.
46. The UCR Time Series Data Mining Archive. (2002). http://www.cs.ucr.edu/~eamonn/TSDMA/index.html.
47. Keogh, E., Xi, X., Wei, L., & Ratanamahatana, C. A. (2006). *The UCR time series classification/clustering homepage.* Retrieved http://www.cs.ucr.edu/~eamonn/time_series_data/.
48. Kiers, H. A. L. (1997). Weighted least squares fitting using ordinary least squares algorithm. *Psychometrika, 62*, 251–266.
49. Kondo, K., Kaneko, T., Baba, M., & Konno, H. (2007). VEGF-C and VEGF-A synergistically enhance lymph node metastasis of gastric cancer. *Biological and Pharmaceutical Bulletin, 30*(4), 633–637.
50. Krzanowski, W. J. (1984). Principal components analysis in the presence of group structure. *Journal of the Royal Statistical Society Series C Applied Statistics, 33*, 164–168.
51. Lebart, L., Morineau, A., & Fénelon, J.P. (1982). *Traitement des données statistiques—méthodes et programmes* (2 Edn). Dunod/BORDAS, Paris.
52. Lerman, I.C., Pinto da Costa, J., & Silva, H. (2002). Validation of very large data sets clustering by means of a nonparametric linear criterion. In K. Jajuga, A. Sokolowski, & H.-H. Bock (Eds.). *Classification, clustering and data analysis. Proceedings of the 8th conference of the International Federation of Classification Societies (IFCS 2002)* (pp. 147–157).
53. Lu, Z., Callan, J. P., & Croft, W. B. (1996). *Measures in collection ranking evaluation.* Technical Report TR96-39, Computer Science Department University of Massachusetts.
54. Medina, P. P., Carretero, J., Fraga, M. F., Esteller, M., Sidransky, D., & Sanchez-Cespedes, M. (2004). Genetic and epigenetic screening for gene alterations of the chromatin-remodeling factor, smarca4/brg1, in lung tumors. *Genes Chromosomes Cancer, 41*(2), 170–177.
55. Mesfioui, M., & Quessy, J.-F. (2010). Concordance measures for multivariate non-continuous random vectors. *Journal of Multivariate Analysis, 101*(10), 2398–2410.
56. Nakhaeizadeh, G., & Schnahl, A. (1998). Development of multi-criteria metrics for evaluation of data mining algorithms. In D. Heckerman, H. Mannila, D. Pregibon & R. Uthurusamy (Eds.), *Proceedings of the fourth international conference on knowledge discovery in databases & data mining* (pp. 37–42). AAAI Press.
57. Neave, H., & Worthington, P. (1992). *Distribution-free tests.* London: Routledge.
58. Nelsen, R. B. (1999). An introduction to copulas. Lecture notes in statistics (Vol. 139). New York: Springer.
59. Nelson, P. T., Baldwin, D. A., Scearce, L. M., Oberholtzer, J. C., Tobias, J. W., & Mourelatos, Z. (2004). Microarray-based, high-throughput gene expression profiling of micrornas. *Nature Methods, 1*, 155–161.
60. Pestana, D., & Velosa, S. (2006). *Introdução à Probabilidade e à Estatística* (Vol. 1). Fundação Calouste Gulbenkian, 2a edição.
61. Pinto da Costa, J. F., Soares, C., & Brazdil, P. (2001). Some improvements in the evaluation of methods to rank alternatives. In *Poster at workshop on non-linear estimation and classification.* Berkeley: MSRI.
62. Pinto da Costa, J. F., & Silva, L. (2003). Feature selection in DNA microarrays. *ACTES Du Xeme Congrès de la Société Francophone de classification (SFC 2003)* (Vol. 10–12, pp. 103–108). Neuchâtel: Suisse.

63. Pinto da Costa, J., & Soares, C. (2005). A weighted rank measure of correlation. *Australian and New Zealand Journal of Statistics*, *47*(4), 515–529.

64. Pinto da Costa, J., Roque, L., & Soares, C. (2015). The weighted rank correlation coefficient r_{W2} in the case of ties. *Statistics and Probability Letters*. doi:10.1016/j.spl.2014.12.024. http://dx.doi.org/10.1016/j.spl.2014.12.024.

65. Pinto da Costa, J., Alonso, H., Roque, L. A. C., & Oliveira, M. M. (2006). Supervised and unsupervised selection of genes in microarray data. In *Proceedings of statistics in genomics and proteomics* (Vol. 27, pp. 65–74). CIM-Centro Internacional de Matemática.

66. Pinto da Costa, J. F., Alonso, H., Roque, L., & Oliveira, M. (2005). Selecting Relevant Genes in Microarray Data. *Poster presented in the Workshop on Statistics in Genomics and Proteomics*. Estoril, Portugal.

67. Pinto da Costa, J., & Roque, L. (2006). Limit distribution for the weighted rank correlation coefficient, r_w. *REVSTAT—Statistical Journal*, *4*(3), 189–200.

68. Pinto da Costa, J., & Soares, C. (2007). Rejoinder to letter to the editor from Genest, C. and Plante, J.F. concerning Pinto da Costa, J. and Soares, C. (2005) A weighted rank measure of correlation. *Australian and New Zealand Journal of Statistics*, *49*(2), 205–207.

69. Pinto da Costa, J., Alonso, H., & Roque, L. (2007). Analysis of gene expression data by PCA and decision trees. In *JOCLAD 2007: XIII Jornadas de Classificação e Análise de Dados*.

70. Pinto da Costa, J., Silva, I., & Silva, M. E. (2007). Time dependent principal component analysis of time series data. In *IASC 07 (book of abstracts): Statistics for data mining, learning and knowledge extraction* (p. 32).

71. Pinto da Costa, J., Silva, I., & Silva, M. E. (2007).Time dependent clustering of time series. In *Bulletin of the International Statistical Institute (ISI 2007): Proceedings of the 56th Session*.

72. Pinto da Costa, J., Alonso, H., & Roque, L. (2009). A weighted principal component analysis and its application to microarray data. In *Proceedings of the conference statistical methods for the analysis of large data-sets, Italian Statistical Society, Coop. Libraria Editrice Universita di Padova* (pp. 203–206). Pescara.

73. Pinto da Costa, J., Alonso, H., & Roque, L. (2011). A weighted principal component analysis and its application to gene expression data. *IEEE/ACM Transactions on Computational Biology and Bioinformatics*, *8*(1), 246–252.

74. Pinto da Costa, J. (2011). Weighted correlation. *International encyclopedia of statistical science* (1st Edn.). LVIII (Vol. 3, p. 1852). ISBN: 978-3-642-04897-5.

75. Pomeroy, S. L., Tamayo, P., Gaasenbeek, M., Sturla, L. M., Angelo, M., McLaughlin, M. E., et al. (2002). Prediction of central nervous system embryonal tumour outcome based on gene expression. *Nature Neuroscience*, *415*, 436–442.

76. Pottier, P. (1994). Mesures de la liaison entre deux variables qualitatives: Relation entre un coefficient de corrélation généralisée et le χ^2. *Revue de Statistique Appliquée*, **XLII**(1), 41–61.

77. Development Core Team, R. (2005). *R: A language and environment for statistical computing*. Vienna, Austria: R Foundation for Statistical Computing.

78. Randles, R. H., & Wolfe, D. A. (1979). Introduction to the theory of nonparametric statistics. *Probability and Mathematical Statistics*. New York: Wiley.

79. Ratanamahatana, C. A., & Keogh. E. (2004). Everything you know about dynamic time warping is wrong. In *Workshop on mining temporal and sequential data, in conjunction with 10th ACM SIGKDD International Conference on Knowledge Discovery and Data Mining*, USA.

80. Roverso, D. (2000). Multivariate temporal classification by windowed wavelet decomposition and recurrent neural networks. In *Proceedings of the 3rd ANS international topical meeting on nuclear plant instrumentation, control and human-machine interface*. USA.

81. Roque, L. (2003). Métodos Inferenciais para o Coeficiente de Correlação ρ_w. Tese de Mestrado em Estatística: Faculdade de Ciências, Universidade do Porto, Portugal.

82. Ripley, B. D. (1996). *Pattern recognition and neural networks*. Cambridge: Cambridge University Press.

83. Ruymgaart, F. H., Shorack, G. R., & Van Zwet, W. R. (1972). Asymptotic normality of nonparametric tests for independence. *The Annals of Mathematical Statistics*, *43*, 1122–1135.

84. Salas, S. L., Hille, E., & Etgen, G. J. (2003). *Calculus: One and several variables* (9th Edn.). New York: Wiley.
85. Sanguinetti, G., Milo, M., Rattray, M., & Lawrence, N. D. (2005). Accounting for probe-level noise in principal component analysis of microarray data. *Bioinformatics, 21,* 3748–3754.
86. Sathyanarayana, U. G., Padar, A., Huang, C. X., Suzuki, M., Shigematsu, H., Bekele, B. N., et al. (2003). Aberrant promoter methylation and silencing of laminin-5-encoding genes in breast carcinoma. *Clinical Cancer Research, 9*(17), 6389–6394.
87. Schafer, J. B., Konstan, J. A., & Riedl, J. (2001). E-commerce recommendation algorithms. *Journal of Data Minig and Knowledge Discovery, 5*(1/2), 115–152.
88. Schmid, F., & Schmidt, R. (2007). Multivariate conditional version of Spearman's rho and related measures of tail dependence. *The Journal of Multivariate Analysis, 98,* 1123–1140.
89. Scholz, M., Gatzek, S., Sterling, A., Fiehn, O., & Selbig, J. (2004). Metabolite fingerprinting: detecting biological features by independent component analysis. *Bioinformatics, 20,* 2447–2454.
90. Slonim, D., Golub, T., Tamayo, P., Mesirov, J. P., & Lander, E. S. (2000). Class prediction and discovery using gene expression data. *RECOMB* (pp. 263–272).
91. Soares, C., Brazdil, P. (2000). Zoomed rankings: Selection of classification algorithms based on relevant performance information. In D. A. Zighed, J. Komorowski & J. Zytkow (Eds.), *Proceedings of the fourth european conference on principles and practice of knowledge discovery in databases (PKDD2000)* (pp. 126–135). Springer.
92. Soares, C., Brazdil, P., & Pinto da Costa, J. (2000). Measures to compare rankings of classification algorithms. In H. Kiers, J.-P. Rasson, P. Groenen & M. Schader (Eds.), *Data analysis, classification and related methods, proceedings of the seventh conference of the International Federation of Classification Societies IFCS* (pp. 119–124). Springer.
93. Soares, C., Pinto da Costa, J., & Brazdil, P. (2001). Improved statistical support for matchmaking: Rank correlation taking rank importance into account. *JOCLAD 2001: VII Jornadas de Classificação e Análise de Dados, Porto, Portugal* (pp. 72–75).
94. Spearman, C. (1904). The proof and measurement of association between two things. *American Journal of Psychology, 15,* 72–101.
95. Speed, T. P. (Ed.). (2003). *Statistical analysis of gene expression microarray data.* London: Chapman and Hall/CRC Press.
96. Terry, J., Saito, T., Subramanian, S., Ruttan, C., Antonescu, C. R., Goldblum, J. R., et al. (2007). TLE1 as a diagnostic immunohistochemical marker for synovial sarcoma emerging from gene expression profiling studies. *The American Journal of Surgical Pathology, 31*(2), 240–246.
97. Tibshirani, R., Hastie, T., Narasimhan, B., & Chu, G. (1999). Diagnosis of multiple cancer types by shrunken centroids of gene expression. *PNAS* (Vol. 10).
98. Tusher, V., Tibshirani, R., & Chu, C. (2001). Significance analysis of microarrays applied to ionizing radiation response. *Proceedings of the national academy of sciences, 98,* 5116–5121.
99. Wang, X., & Smith, K. (2006). Characteristic-based clustering for time series data. *Data Mining and Knowledge Discovery, 13*(3), 335–364.
100. Wold, H., & Lyttkens, E. (1969). Nonlinear iterative partial least squares (NIPALS) estimation procedures. In *Bulletin of the international statistical institute: Proceedings of the 37th session* (pp. 1–15).
101. Xu, X., Yamamoto, H., Sakon, M., Yasui, M., Ngan, C. Y., Fukunaga, H., et al. (2003). Overexpression of CDC25A phosphatase is associated with hypergrowth activity and poor prognosis of human hepatocellular carcinomas. *Clinical Cancer Research, 9*(5), 1764–1772.
102. Yu, T., & Li, K. C. (2005). Inference of transcriptional regulatory network by two-stage constrained space factor analysis. *Bioinformatics, 21,* 4033–4038.
103. Yunta, M., & Lazo, P. A. (2003). Apoptosis protection and survival signal by the CD53 tetraspanin antigen. *Oncogene, 22*(8), 1219–1224.

Printed in the United States
By Bookmasters